STUDIES IN EXISTENTIALISM
AND PHENOMENOLOGY

Editor: R. D. Laing

Psychiatry and Anti-Psychiatry

Psychiatry
and
Anti-Psychiatry

David G. Cooper

III

TAVISTOCK PUBLICATIONS
LONDON, NEW YORK, SYDNEY, TORONTO, WELLINGTON

First published in 1967
by Tavistock Publications Limited
11 New Fetter Lane, London E.C.4

This book is set in 12 point Bembo
and was printed in Great Britain by
The Camelot Press Ltd, Southampton

Distributed in the U.S.A.
by Barnes & Noble, Inc.

To the memory
of my father

Contents

	Preface	ix
	Introduction	I
I	Violence and Psychiatry	14
II	Families and Schizophrenia	34
III	Studying One Family	46
IV	The Invalid, his Family, and the Ward	73
V	Villa 21 – An Experiment in Anti-Psychiatry	83
VI	Furthermore	105
	Appendix The Question of Results: An Ironic Addendum	112
	References	127

Preface

For anyone who works in the psychiatric field and who refuses to allow his critical awareness of what he is about to be numbed or engulfed by the institutionalizing processes of formal training and day-by-day indoctrination in the teaching hospital or psychiatric hospital, a number of disturbing questions arise. In this field most particularly, in the midst of people in extreme situations, one experiences the Zen 'doubt sensation' – why am I here, who put me here, or why have I put myself here (and what is the difference between these questions), who is paying me for what, what shall I do, why do anything, why do nothing, what is anything and what is nothing, what is life and death, sanity and madness?

To the institutional survivor none of the more or less glib customary answers to these questions seems adequate. The questioning extends into both the theoretical basis, such as it is, of one's work and the precise daily operations—gestures, acts, statements in relation to actual other persons. A more profound questioning has led some of us to propose conceptions and procedures that seem quite antithetic to the conventional ones – in fact what may be regarded as a germinal anti-psychiatry.

The most effective way to explore the possibilities of such an antithetic discipline seems to me to be to investigate the major problem area of the discipline in question. In the case of psychiatry this problem area is that which is defined as schizophrenia.

What I have attempted to do in this monograph is to take a look at the person who has been labelled schizophrenic in his actual human context and to enquire how this label came to be attached to him, by whom it was attached, and what it signifies both for the labellers and the labelled.

This is a study of one mode of social invalidation, but it takes this term in a dual sense. First, a person is progressively made to conform to the inert, passive identity of invalid or patient – although part of this identity implies that he produces the illusion of activity, for example in occupation departments of the institution, on the sports fields, and so on. Prior to, concurrently with, and dialectically linked to invalidation in this sense is, second, the process whereby almost every act, statement, and experience of the labelled person is systematically ruled invalid according to certain rules of the game established by his family, and later by others, in their efforts to produce the vitally needed invalid-patient. We shall have to examine these 'vital needs'.

Over the last century psychiatry, in the view of an increasing number of present-day psychiatrists, has aligned itself far too closely with the alienated needs of the society within which it functions. In doing so it is perpetually in danger of committing a well-intentioned act of betrayal of those members of society who have been ejected into the psychiatric situation as patients. A great many people today in this country of their own accord go to their doctors seeking psychiatric help. For the most part such people in very practical terms are seeking the gift of a set of techniques that would enable them all the better and more closely to conform with massified social expectations. They are usually assisted towards this goal. A few misguided persons go to the psychiatrist seeking what amounts to a form of spiritual guidance. They are usually rapidly disillusioned.

Most of the people about whom I shall be writing in this volume, however, have been precipitated into the psychiatric situation by others, usually their families. The fact that most of them these days have the legal status of informal rather than detained patients is merely an ironic incidental note as far as this argument is concerned. They are mostly young people, in their first or second admission to the mental hospital, who have acquired the very specific label 'schizophrenic'. It is people with this label who occupy two-thirds of the beds in most mental hospitals, and we must recall that nearly half the total hospital beds in the

United Kingdom are mental-hospital beds. Nearly 1 per cent of the population at some time in their lives are hospitalized with what is called a 'schizophrenic breakdown', and the celebrated Swiss psychiatrist, E. Bleuler, once said that for every hospitalized schizophrenic there were ten in the community. But then if we look at the statistics in this way we are already prejudging schizophrenia as some sort of actual entity which some people 'have'. And here we would begin to err.

In our society there are many techniques by which certain minorities are first so designated and then dealt with along a continuum of operations running from insinuated derogation, black-balling from certain clubs, exclusion from certain schools and certain jobs, and so on, through total invalidation as persons, bumping off, and mass extermination, at the remoter end of the continuum. Public conscience is, however, so strong, that it demands an excuse for such actions; and the excuse is provided by the prior exercise of techniques of invalidation that are aimed at providing a quantity of ready victims for the actual eliminative procedures.

There is no technique of invalidation more respectable, or even sacrosanct, than that which has the blessing of medical science. Medicine, although always a little upper-class-conscious and stuffy, is traditionally liberal and humane. It has high ideals and the Hippocratic Oath. Psychiatry, although some of its practitioners have begun to strain on the leash, is part of medicine. We shall have occasion, however, in these pages to question the appropriateness of medical or pseudo-medical ways of seeing things and of acting in the field of human behaviour with which psychiatry concerns itself. We shall, in fact, have to consider the point of view that psychiatry, over a major area of its whole field of operation, has been co-operating in the systematic invalidation of a wide category of persons.

I have, first, proposed an orientation with respect to the schizophrenia problem that differs significantly from the conventional clinical approach but relates itself to some of the family studies, carried out in the United States, which I have summarized in Chapter II, and more specifically to the phenomenological family studies of R. D. Laing and A. Esterson in the United Kingdom.

The third chapter seeks paradigmatically to make intelligible the patient-career of one young diagnosed schizophrenic in terms of the nature of his family world and the key events that have happened in it. My experience is that the intelligibility that can be demonstrated in this case is present in most of the others, and that, to say the least, one cannot assume ever that one is dealing with a set of opaque clinical data, that is to say data which may be (at least theoretically) biologically explicable but which are socially unintelligible.

In the fourth and fifth chapters I have outlined the principles and practice of an experimental therapeutic unit for young schizophrenic patients, within a large mental hospital, in which I have referred to the problem of institutional irrationality (as distinct from the irrationality of patients) and the difficulties this creates for the type of social psychiatric experimentation that I feel to be necessary and have sought to justify. I believe that it is only in such a unit that we can explore the possibility of arriving at a non-exploitative, non-invalidating strategy for dealing with people who are admitted to hospital because they are said to be mad. Although this unit shared many of the ideas of 'therapeutic community' as put forward by Maxwell Jones, Wilmer, Artiss, and others, it was, I believe, unique in so far as it dealt with schizophrenic patients according to a 'family-orientated' therapeutic ideology.

Above all, I have been concerned with the question of violence in psychiatry and have concluded that perhaps the most striking form of violence in psychiatry is nothing less than the violence *of* psychiatry in so far as this discipline chooses to refract and condense on to its identified patients the subtle violence of the society it only too often represents to and against these patients. I have envisaged a future experimental unit in which work based on this realization may be furthered.

Some of the text, especially the introduction, is necessarily complex and 'technical' but I hope that the reader will find it worth while to struggle through such stretches. To express the content more readably may be possible, but the complexity is unavoidable because it reflects the real complexity of real human events.[1]

I am deeply indebted above all to Dr R. D. Laing and Dr A. Esterson at every level of my writing in this book, but they bear no responsibility for what I have said. I would like to thank the Medical Advisory Committee and the Management Committee of the hospital concerned for facilities to carry out my work and in particular the consultant-in-charge, Dr S. T. Hayward. The Research Sub-Committee of the Regional Hospital Board responsible kindly provided money for secretarial assistance in my family research work. Dr J. D. Sutherland read most of the manuscript of the book and made helpful criticisms. I am also grateful to Dr J. Humphrey, Dr J. Macintyre, and Mr Paul Senft for either practical help in my project or reading portions of manuscript. I would stress again, however, that none of these people or bodies bears any responsibility for the views I have expressed here; some of them in fact have expressed considerable difference of opinion.

Above all I am indebted to all the people who have lived and worked in the unit in Villa 21.

Acknowledgements

Thanks are due to Heinemann and Company for permission to quote the passage from *The Prophet* by Kahlil Gibran (1926 edition, reprinted 1965), and to the Editor of the *British Medical Journal* for permission to use in the Appendix the article entitled 'Results of family-orientated therapy with hospitalized schizophrenics' (*Brit. med. J.*, 18 December 1965 (2), 1462–5).

---

[1] For a more detailed introduction to some of the key concepts used in this book I would refer the reader to R. D. Laing and D. G. Cooper, *Reason and violence* (1964).

Introduction

On est toujours libre de ne rien comprendre à rien. Gabriel Marcel

If we take the most recent segment of psychiatric history, say the last ten to fifteen years, we find that approaches to what is called schizophrenia fall into two general categories. On the one hand there are the conventional approaches which claim or, more usually, assume without feeling the need to claim, that there is a nosological (i.e. disease-classificatory) entity called schizophrenia which has to be accounted for causally. On the other hand there is the approach which points out that a disease entity has by no means been firmly established and that the disease 'model', or way of thinking, is perhaps not the most appropriate with which to approach the 'schizophrenia field',[1] or that, even, it is a model totally at odds with the very nature of this field.

The quasi-medical nosological approach assumes that, since it is dealing with a disease, there are symptoms and signs that may be observed in an objectifiable person who may be (implicitly or explicitly) abstracted from his human environment for the purpose of making such observations, and, further, that the symptoms and signs indicate a diagnosis that, in turn, indicates prognosis and treatment. This supposed diagnostic entity must by definition have a cause; and here views diverge, although with remarkably little evidential basis, between biochemical abnormality, virus infection, structural fault in the brain, constitutional-genetic origin (which may be related to other causes), and psychological causation.

The other approach, to which it is not yet easy to attach a label,

[1] As I shall term that social field where the label schizophrenia is attached by some participants in the field to other participants.

I

tends to regard 'schizophrenia' as a bad attack of what Wittgenstein called 'the bewitchment of our intelligence by language'. The American psychiatrist T. S. Szasz applies the term *panchreston* to schizophrenia. A panchreston is an 'explain-all', rather like the 'cure-all', 'broad-spectrum psychotropic' drugs. In fact, it is suggested, the term schizophrenia has done little but confuse the real problem, and there is not one shred of unequivocally credible evidence to support the inclusion of schizophrenia as a disease-entity in the field of medical nosology.

Schizophrenia, however, is not an entirely meaningless term for workers of this latter orientation, and I would provide the following tentative definition to guide our inquiry: *schizophrenia is a micro-social[1] crisis situation in which the acts and experience of a certain person are invalidated by others for certain intelligible cultural and micro-cultural (usually familial) reasons, to the point where he is elected and identified as being 'mentally ill' in a certain way, and is then confirmed (by a specifiable but highly arbitrary labelling process) in the identity 'schizophrenic patient' by medical or quasi medical agents.* This statement, it will be noted, refers to extreme disturbance (crisis) in a group and says nothing about disorder in a 'schizophrenic' person. The elected person, however, has usually, prior to the crisis, grown up to experience the world in a manner conditioned by a global or partial lack of consensual validation of his self- and other-perception. The resultant experiential and behavioural state is sometimes referred to by psychiatrists as 'schizoid'. Here again I assume no primary defect in the patient-to-be but would suggest that there is a demonstrable failure in a micro-social field of persons in relation.

With this definitional statement as our point of departure, the central problem, as I see it, is to take the behavioural picture, the totality of verbal and non-verbal communicative behaviour presented by the diagnosed 'acute schizophrenic patient' around the time of his admission to the reception unit, and then to discover to what extent this picture is intelligible in terms of what

[1] The term *micro-social* refers to a finite group of persons in face-to-face interaction – persons who look at, and are looked at by, each other

has gone on and what is going on between the patient and the other persons to whom he stands in relation. I shall, in pursuing this intelligibility, focus particularly on the patient's family since in the case of young patients on their first admission the family are usually the most actively significant other persons with whom the patient is currently involved.

The heuristic value of this way of stating the problem has been suggested by experiences gathered in talking to schizophrenic patients, their families, and then the patients seen together with their families. The latter type of interview, to which the way was pointed by a growing body of family studies in the United States, produces a highly specific kind of group-interactional situation and it is from experience in this situation that the hypothetical formulations presented in this monograph have primarily developed.

I decided that concurrently with observations on the patient's interaction in the ward group the patients would be seen separately with their families. These two group interactions would then be compared, with a view to ascertaining what light could be thrown on phenomena in the ward interaction by the understanding we developed of the functioning of the family group.

Immediate objections are raised when an investigation of this nature is proposed: Where are your controls? How are you going to quantify any of your material? How can you claim any generality for your statements on the basis of only a small number of cases? What we have to recognize on hearing these objections is that there are certain natural-scientific principles which have been imported without qualification by some workers into the field of the sciences of persons (or anthropological sciences) and have then been proclaimed as desiderata if not first essentials or preconditions of any study that would call itself scientific. This tendency has led to endless methodological confusion and repeated attempts to prove things in terms in which 'proof' is an *a priori* impossibility in this field.

I shall digress from the narrower issue of schizophrenia at this point and consider somewhat schematically the stages through which experimental natural science proceeds and then go on to consider the applicability or relevance of each stage to a 'science of persons'. Perhaps it is only in terms of such a scientific framework that we shall be able to make sense of what seems to be madness.

Experimental natural science is grounded in careful observation. Each investigation must proceed from observed facts. In physical and biological science these observed facts are usually *inert* facts, that is to say they are grasped from the exterior by an observer who is not disturbed by them and does not disturb them by his process of observation. Even in micro-physics where the uncertainty principle tells us that the observational procedures disturb the field of the observed, there are mathematical techniques which maintain the observer in some sort of relation of exteriority to the observed and indeed to his observing techniques themselves. In a science of personal interaction, on the other hand, mutual disturbance of the observer and the observed is not only inevitable in every case *but it is this mutual disturbance which gives rise to the primary facts on which theory is based*, and not the disturbed or disturbing personal entities. The facts that constitute the observational data of anthropological sciences are not different from the facts from which natural science proceeds in the same sense that facts for biology are different from facts for physics: they differ *in ontological status* from natural-scientific facts. Put another way, the observer-observed relation in a science of persons in ontologically continuous (subject-object *vis-à-vis* subject-object), whereas in natural sciences it is discontinuous (subject *vis-à-vis* object) permitting a purely exterior description of the field of the observed.

From statements of observed fact, the natural scientist proceeds to conjectural statements that assume the conditional form, 'if such and such conditions obtain, we may expect so and so in the observational field'. If these predictions expressed in the hypothesis are experimentally verified we are in a position to form a theory. In the sphere of personal action, however, conditional statements are complicated in this way: given these specifiable conditions we may expect this person, on the basis of everything we know about him and his past, to behave in this particular way; however, personal action in its essence is the possibility of 'depassing'[1] all determinations of what it is to be and proceeding perhaps in the direction opposite to that expected – unless there is a locatable choice to conform with such expectations, a choice not to choose. Certainly the field of human actions is readily seen in probabilistic terms but what cannot be left out of the question is the possibility of the subject's realizing this probabilistic structuring of the field in which he is situated and, through this realization, destructuring the field and acting 'improbably'. This possibility, which the subject always has, of altering his conduct from the expected, through reflective awareness of the factors that are conditioning him at a certain time, really constitutes a crucial difference.

In short, while we are entitled to, and in any practical context must have, *expectations* (which we must expect to be disappointed) about a person's behaviour, natural-scientific *prediction* must be seen to be neither possible nor impossible in the sciences of persons but simply inappropriate to the field of discourse.

In the natural sciences verifiability and falsifiability of hypotheses depend on the *repeatability* of situations. In the sciences of persons, however, we note that repetition of an individual or group life-historical situation is in principle impossible. There are certainly all the appearances of repetition but in each case we discover that this 'repetition' is the product of an illusory project of self-dehistoricization. A person dehistoricizes himself when he chooses (however unknowingly) to deny that by a prior series of choices he has moved his life on from an earlier situation to a new situation: this denial (an act which, by a further act, he denies in turn and so 'does not know') allows an illusion of a historical fixity and substantiality. This is the principal mode in which a

---

[1] To depass: a transliteration of the French term *dépasser* as used by J.-P. Sartre in *Critique de la raison dialectique* (1960). It should be understood in the sense of Hegel's *aufheben*, i.e. movement beyond the existing state of affairs to a further state, or synthesis, which conserves the earlier state in a modified form in a new totalization.

person rids himself of the anxiety that issues from a recognition of his responsibility for himself. It is remarkable to find scientific theory sometimes effecting the same evasion.

If repetition of life-historical situations is impossible, then natural-scientific criteria of verifiability and falsifiability of hypotheses become irrelevant and we must find other criteria by which we may know that we are speaking 'the truth'. To do this we have to distinguish between two types of rationality, each appropriate to a field of discourse different from, but inter-related with, that of the other. These types we call analytical and dialectical rationality.

By analytical rationality I mean a logic of exteriority according to which truth lies, according to certain criteria, in propositions formed outside the reality with which they are concerned. The epistemological model here is characterized by a dual passivity: the observed system is passive with respect to the observer (what-ever actions and reactions go on within the system); the observer is passive in relation to the system he observes; such activity as he appears to manifest being limited to conceptual rearrangements of the facts, which are registered on him from the outside, and to inferences he makes from these facts.

This type of rationality has a valid field of application in, for example, classical physics, where the objects of science are inert totalities, but its transportation into the fields of psychology, sociology, and history is another matter, for here its validity is severely restricted. Human reality is that sector of reality where *totalization* is the very mode of being. A totality is something completed, which therefore can be grasped as a whole; a totaliza-tion, on the other hand, is a perpetual movement, throughout the life of a subject – a movement of progressive synthetic self-definition, and this cannot in principle be grasped by a method that would arrest it. Analytical rationality involves the assump-tion of a perspective of complete exteriority in this sense: I sum you up, that is I grasp you conceptually as a totality, and that is all there is to it. But if, simultaneously with my summing-up of you, you sum me up, I have to include your summing-up of me in my summing-up of you. That is to say, the situation becomes more complex in a most specific way. What goes on in the reciprocal relation of a two-person transaction is as follows: I totalize you but you, in your reciprocal totalization of me, include my totalization of you, so that my totalization of you involves a totalization of your totalization of me, and so on. In the transaction each of us is a moving synthetic unity of totalization-detotalization. With every act I objectify myself, I imprint myself on the world, and this objectification of myself issues from the totalization-in-process that I am. But my objectification of myself escapes my sphere of control and enters yours so that you may interpret my actions as having a significance totally different from that which I intend. I freely produce an impression of myself in the world, but this very free act produces an objectification by which you, through your freedom, limit my freedom. Similarly I, through my freedom, limit yours.

This view of human relations is made clear in the following example:[1] I am surreptitiously looking through a keyhole at an intimate scene in the next room. I become aware of a presence behind me. I turn and discover that someone has been watching me. At that moment a 'haemorrhage' occurs. The pure subjectivity that I have been existing as an observer of the scene in the next room drains away from my world into the world of the other where I become nothing more than a shameful object observed by him – at least, until I find a way to regain my existence, return to the centre of *my* world, and reduce the other in turn to being an object for me. It is the dialectic between accepting the periphery and seizing the centre.

What I have described here as a reciprocal relation is a relation of interiority, but in addition these two persons are organismal realities linked to each other by a relation of exteriority. Anatomical and physiological descriptions of a person's body deal with the person as a 'pure object' in relation to which the biological scientist adopts a purely exterior perspective. While this exterior

[1] Essentially on the lines of the example quoted by Sartre in *Being and nothingness* (1957, Part III, Chapter IV).

7

perspective accords with certain conventional ideas of scientific objectivity, its limits are very closely drawn. These limits, when we discover them, reveal the extent to which, say, biochemical theories of the cause of schizophrenia must *of necessity* (however far biochemical technique may advance) fall short of their stated goal of causal explanation.

The implicit rationality of such causalistic theories, which we term analytic rationality, excludes by definition any comprehension of relations of interiority between persons (sometimes called intersubjectivity) and yet it is such relations that mediate the series of acts which we call 'schizophrenic behaviour', that is to say, the way in which the labelled schizophrenic person objectifies himself in the world. If we are to comprehend this mediation, if we are to discover the intelligibility of schizophrenic behaviour, or any other sort of behaviour, we require not merely some special descriptive technique but a type of rationality radically distinct from the analytic rationality of natural science. This other type of rationality is dialectical rationality.

Dialectical rationality is concrete in the sense that it is nothing more than its actual functioning in the world of actual entities. It is a method of knowing in which by knowing we understand the grasping of intelligible structures *in their intelligibility*. In these terms we comprehend dialectical rationality as comprehensive: it must not only know objects but must, in the same act, constitute its own criteria for the (dialectical) truth of its assertions about these objects. Dialectical knowledge of objects is inextricable from knowledge of dialectical knowledge and both are necessary moments in a synthetic process which we call the dialectic. But the dialectic is not only an epistemological principle, a principle of knowing about knowing, but also an ontological principle, a principle of knowing about being. There is a certain sector of reality, a whole group of actual entities, which we know and in which there is a movement that is dialectic. Dialectic then is both a method of knowing and a movement in the object known. This movement is not the inert *process* studied by natural scientific disciplines but *praxis*, that is to say totalizing activity which is not simply constituted by a field of real events, but which constitutes itself as a certain mode of being and constitutes a certain field of other entities in a certain relation to itself. This sector of reality is *human reality* and its scientific study is anthropology, understood as a science of persons. Anthropology so conceived forms the meta-theory for a number of disciplines – psychology, micro-sociology, sociology, social anthropology – into each of which in various ways historiography is absorbed in so far as this latter is more than a mere chronological record. Historiography, then, is distinct from history, which is an actual activity of the persons with which historiographical study concerns itself. History is what men, all men, do and have done.[1]

The dialectic is a totalizing activity in which two types of unification are related: the unifying unification (the act of knowing) and the unified unification (the object known). Human action and interaction and their social products are *intelligible* if we can trace in them a pattern of synthesis of a multiplicity into a whole. If we are able to take a further step and link praxis (acts of an individual or group) to an intention of an individual or group, then we have discovered the *comprehensibility* of the praxis. If, however, through alienation, act has become divorced from intention we may still discover the intelligibility of the act though it is incomprehensible. The effect of this divorce of act from intention is amply exemplified in political life, where political figures carry out pseudo-acts, make pseudo-decisions, and produce pseudo-events according to the intentions of more or less anonymous pressure groups and backroom advisers. In large institutions such as mental hospitals, an obscure praxis floats between various levels of the hierarchy and then, without an obvious identifiable agent, obstructs or furthers a certain organizational change.

In the families of schizophrenic patients intentions that link up with the 'psychotic acts' of the patient are denied or, even, their antitheses are asserted in such a way that the patient's actions have

---

[1] Cf. Marx, 'History is *nothing* but the activity of men in pursuit of their ends' (Marx-Engels *Gesamtausgabe*, Vol. 1, Section 3, p. 265).

the appearance of pure process unrelated to praxis and may even be experienced by him as such.

When things reach this pass the identified patient must, in order to achieve some coherence in his world view, some 'sanity', imaginatively invent a representation of these mysterious influences that act on him. This is where 'delusions' of influence by people from outer space or another planet, or even more local institutions such as the Catholic Church, the Communist Party, or the Freemasons, find their real meaning.

The patient thus seeks to render more intelligible the actual happenings between him and others, but the only ways in which he may do this have previously been ruled to be 'delusional' by the rest of his society. It is ironic that if we seek intelligibility hard enough, we run the risk of being thought mad or of being in some other way dismissed or invalidated.

Reductive analyses, whether these be framed in terms of physiology, learning theory, or psycho-analytic theory, may very competently and in detail portray the extra- and intra-organismal background against which the person stands, but in each case, and for the same reason, the personal reality itself is omitted. In each case the reductive approaches we have mentioned end in a specifically interrelated aggregate of inert totalities – neuro-physiological or biochemical mechanisms, instinctive units of behaviour, libidinal and aggressive drives. The passively produced point of intersection of a series of abstract theoretical lines is proposed as the (more or less) irreducible reality of the person. All this is not only beside the point when we question a personal reality, it is a point about something else entirely. Reductive analyses consist of statements about the way in which a personal entity is constituted by means of factors that are exterior to it (even when the factors are forces within the person's body, they are exterior in the sense of being within his body as an object for another and not the body which he exists).[1] Personal life, however, is not only constituted from the exterior but *constitutes*

[1] See Sartre's well-known description of the body in *Being and nothingness* (1957, Part 3, Chapter 2).

itself on the basis of this exterior constitution of it. Put another way, the person chooses himself on the basis of (against, in the face of, or in compliance with) the totality of factors that condition him.

These considerations give us the clue to a more adequate schema that would provide the meta-theoretical, meta-methodological basis for theories about the lives of persons and hypotheses regarding transactions between persons from the level of the small group to that of history. Such a schema must be progressive as well as regressive, synthetic as well as analytic, for, while the historical movement of a person's life in relation to the lives of other persons consists of a series of analysable 'moments' and relations between moments, it is in its very essence a synthesis in progress, a moving unity, a totalization perpetually retotalizing itself on the basis of its interiorization of its detotalization by others.

There are, first, the acts by which a person presents himself to us; in these acts we trace an intention or intentions that relate to a prior and more basic choice of self: this presentation of self, which is pure flux perpetually exceeding its perpetual objectification of itself in the world, is the *constituted dialectic*.[1] From a phenomenological description of this constituted moment we proceed by a *regressive movement* to a *constitutive dialectic*: by this latter term we mean all the socio-environmental (intra-familial, extra-familial, economic-class, social-historical) conditioning factors in their inter-penetrating fullness. But we cannot end here. By a *progressive movement* we must attain the personal synthesis, the total totalization – the person's unique totalization of the conditioning totalization on the basis of its totalization of him. We have then attained the 'truth' of the person's life, or of some specific sector of his life.

In other words, we have to trace what the person does with

---

[1] The pairs of terms, constitutive/constituted and progressive/regressive are taken from Sartre's *Critique de la raison dialectique*.

For an exposition of these terms in English see R. D. Laing and D. G. Cooper, *Reason and violence* (1964, pp. 95 and 49 ff respectively).

what is done to him, what he makes of what he is made of. Each of these terms, 'what he does', 'what is done to him', 'what he is made of', can individually be the object of an analytic investigation. But they are nothing more than 'moments'. That is to say they are terms in opposition to other terms in a dialectic, which can only be isolated at the price of distortion of the rest of the total picture.

If in dealing with persons acting in relation to each other, we are dealing with synthetic unities, and if the central 'schizophrenia problem' is posed in terms of persons acting in relation, then we are patently operating on a level beyond reduction to a quantitative formalism. We then recognize how illusory is the view that general statements must, at least ideally, assume the form of quantitative mathematical expressions. To say this by no means precludes the expression of general statements concerning personal interaction in a formal language – on the contrary, I believe that the working-out of a non-metric, relational formalism is a clear possibility and one that must be pursued.[1]

Finally, on the issue of generalization from a small series, when it is objected that the limited number of cases may be special and unrepresentative cases, one could not do better than recall the words of Kurt Goldstein (1951, p. 25):

'This objection completely misunderstands the real situation ... an accumulation of facts even numerous is of no help if these facts were imperfectly established; it does not lead to the knowledge of things as they really happen. ... We must choose only these cases which permit of formulating final judgements. And then what is true for one case will also be true for any other.'

[1] See C. Lévi-Strauss's article 'On social structure' (1953, pp. 524–33). Lévi-Strauss points out that there is no necessary connection between social structure and measure although one may be able to assign numerical values to certain invariants, e.g. in Kroeber's studies of women's dress fashions. There may, however, be a rigorous non-metric mathematical approach, perhaps using existing techniques of mathematical logic, set theory, group theory, and topology. I would remind the reader here, however, that Kurt Lewin's work with topological constructs is not such a relational formalism in so far as he deploys metric vectors in his topological fields.

In other words, what may falsely be construed as bias may in fact be judicious selection. The criteria for judicious selection in this field must be the subject for a further work, but for the moment let us establish this principle, digest it, assimilate it, realize it in its entirety of implication, and get on with the work we have to do.

The work we have to do concerns madness. It concerns that most representative area of madness to which doctors and even scientists have accorded the label schizophrenia. Whether or not the disease schizophrenia exists we shall have to discuss and dispute, but beyond this zone of uncertainty lies an area of certainty. I am quite sure, and shall give some of the reasons for my certitude, that the process whereby someone becomes a designated schizophrenic involves a subtle, psychological, mythical, mystical, spiritual violence. This violence is so devious that it has eluded its inexorable pinning-down for at least the last century, but now finally we may be able to begin to say what it is.

This investigation must lead us on to a consideration of more basic structures and these structures will involve us in an examination of the family and, in particular, the ways in which the family mediates a general social alienation and estrangement to all its members, but most crucially and destructively to its young.

Having, I hope, disabused ourselves of the prevalent pseudo-scientism, let us prod our divining-rod, with an excusable rhetorical flourish, into the innards of the violence that people do to each other.

CHAPTER I

Violence and Psychiatry

At the heart of our problem is violence. The sort of violence that I shall consider here, however, has little to do with people hitting each other on the head with hammers and will not much be about what crazy mental patients are supposed to do. If one is to speak of violence in psychiatry, the violence that stares out screaming, proclaiming itself as such so loudly that it is rarely heard, is the subtle, tortuous violence that other people, the 'sane ones', perpetrate against the labelled madmen. In so far as psychiatry represents the interests or pretended interests of the sane ones, we may discover that, in fact, violence in psychiatry is pre-eminently the violence *of* psychiatry.

But who are these sane people? How do they define themselves? Definitions of mental health propounded by the experts usually amount to the notion of conformism to a set of more or less arbitrarily posited social norms, or else they are so conveniently general – for example, 'the capacity to tolerate and develop through conflict' – that they deprive themselves of operational significance. One is left with the sorry reflection that the sane ones are perhaps those who fail to gain admission to the mental observation ward. That is to say, they define themselves by a certain absence of experience. But then the Nazis gassed tens of thousands of mental patients, and tens of thousands more in this country have their brains surgically mutilated or battered by successive courses of electro-shock and, above all, their personalities systematically deformed by psychiatric institutionalization.

How can such very concrete facts emerge on the basis of an absence, a negativity – the compulsive non-madness of the sane?

In fact, this whole area of definition of sanity and madness is so confused and those who venture into it so uniformly terrified (whether they are 'professionally qualified' or not) by the hint of what they might encounter, not only in 'the others' but also in themselves, that one must seriously consider relinquishing the project. One cannot proceed, I believe, without challenging the basic classification of clinical psychiatry of people into 'psychotic', 'neurotic', and 'normal'. But then, since the history of psychiatry has consisted very largely in the elaboration of an immense public convenience that takes the form of large mental hospitals, outpatient clinics, general-hospital psychiatric units, and, sometimes, unfortunately, the psycho-analytic couch, one should not let this deter one from attempting what might seem to be a radical and possibly dangerous re-evaluation of the problem of madness.

The essence of this necessary re-evaluation of madness, as I see it, is perhaps most aptly and economically expressed in the diagram (*Figure 1*). In this schematic representation, which for present purposes restricts itself to a very conventional terminology, we discover first the point of insertion of the individual person at point alpha. From this point the person develops in the sense of progressively taking into himself, registering, and then acting on the things his parents are taught, feel, and then teach him to be the 'correct' things. Along with this he learns his 'masculine-instrumental' or she learns her 'feminine-expressive' social role. If all progresses 'well' in his family and school, he attains the point of adolescent 'identity crisis' where he, in effect, sums up everything that has conditioned him so far, all the early identifications he has made, all the things that he has been 'made of', everything he has been stuffed full of. (This constitutes 'normality' – a statistical concept that most of us live by as a golden rule.) Then, more or less successfully, he projects himself into an independent future, but one which must of necessity, unless there has been some fortunate error, reduce him to what is conventionally accepted. From this point on he lives forty or fifty years in what remains virtually the same state, although by a process of accretion he becomes more 'experienced', 'wise', develops a greater capacity to adjust to altering circumstances, knows what is 'best' for him and probably for most other people. He lives in this way and then dies. He is known, remembered, and then forgotten. These latter periods may vary chronologically

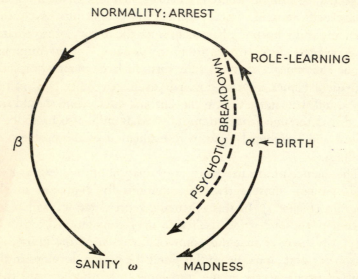

Figure 1

From the moment of birth most people progress through the social learning situations of family and school until they achieve social normality. Most people are developmentally arrested in this state of normality. Some others break down during this progress and regress to what is called madness in the diagram. Others, very few, manage to slip through the state of inertia or arrest represented by alienated, statistical normality and progress to some extent on the way (β) to sanity, retaining an awareness of the criteria of social normality so that they may avoid invalidation (this is always a dicey game). One should note that normality is 'far out' at an opposite pole not only to madness but also to sanity. Sanity approaches madness but an all-important gap, a difference, always remains. This is the omega point (ω).

but on the cosmic time-scale they do not matter at all. This is surely the career and the fate of most of us, particularly if we are 'mentally healthy'.

Perhaps, however, this need not be so. Perhaps there is some manner in which we may escape or liberate ourselves into a more real, less stereotyped future. I think there is, but then one runs the risk of being thought mad and one is then in danger of psychiatric treatment. Psychiatric treatment is often ridiculed in terms of its failure, but this is most unjust. If one is to speak truly of the failure of psychiatric treatment one must be prepared to see that its failure resides most precisely in its success. This treatment in either its official or unofficial guise (non-medical therapeutic conditioning) usually succeeds in producing a requisite conformism either on the level of the chronic back ward or on the (higher or lower) level of the all-commanding captain of industry. There are many species and genera of vegetables but all of them, by our principles of classification, lie in the mud. They grow there and they are gathered there. Potatoes, Tomatoes, Chicory, and Turnips. Non-human ones and human ones. To alter the analogy, one might say that we live lives that are boxed in[1] from birth to death. From the womb we are born into the box of the family from which we progress into the box of the school. By the time we leave school we have become so conditioned to being in a box that from then on we erect our own box, prison, bin around us—until, finally with relief, we are put into the coffin or the oven. I shall return later in this volume to the prospect of liberation but in the meantime there are other tasks. Let us simply note the possible connection between socially prescribed sanity, psychiatric treatment, and boxes.

We must look at the Sane a little more closely. Despairing of connotation, we see that denotatively they include the families of the patients, employers at work, general practitioners, mental welfare officers, the police, magistrates, social workers, psychiatrists, mental nurses, and many others. All these people, some of

[1] Compare Pete Seeger's well-known folk-song 'Little Boxes, on the Hillside'; this expresses very well the nature of the 'boxed-in' condition.

17

whom may be most sincere and devoted to the patient, are implicated more or less deeply, but inexorably albeit despite themselves, in a subtle violence against the objects of their care. I do not have the intention of denigrating certain psychiatrists and other mental health workers who are struggling quite genuinely, and often against formidable institutional obstacles, to provide authentic help for their patients. But, of course, we have also to remember that good intentions and all the trappings of professional respectability very often cover a truly cruel human reality. We recall, for instance, that Boger of Auschwitz had ideas for dealing with teenage delinquents not dissimilar from those expressed by many respected and eminent members of *our* society, and that Dr Capesius has been noted since the war to be particularly considerate and kindly towards animals and children.

To comprehend my present usage of the term 'violence', we shall have to understand it as the corrosive action of the freedom of a person on the freedom of another. It is not direct physical assaultiveness, although this may issue from it. The free action (or praxis) of a person can destroy the freedom of another or at least paralyse it by mystification. Human groups are formed in relation to some real or illusory menace outside the group, but as this external menace becomes more remote, the group, which has literally or metaphorically become a pledged group, is faced with the necessity to reinvent fear to ensure its own permanence.[1] This secondary fear, which is a free product of the group determined to prevent its internal dissolution, is *terror* induced by the *violence* of common freedom. Violence in this sense, in the psychiatric field, commences in the family of the mental patient-to-be. But it does not end there.

---

[1] The pledged group displays a form of reciprocity that Sartre has called the pledge (*serment*). A multiplicity of freedoms produce a common praxis aimed at securing some basis for permanence of the group. The resulting form of reciprocity is the pledge. Only occasionally is this reciprocity expressed in words or ritual acts.

The original account of this is in Sartre, *Critique de la raison dialectique* (1960). An exposition in English is available in R. D. Laing and D. G. Cooper, *Reason and violence* (1964, Part 3, pp. 129 ff.).

In the mental hospital there are people with widely differing problems. In some cases behaviour that is regarded socially as disturbed is explicable in terms of biological processes such as brain disease, pathological ageing of the brain, epilepsy and so on. But in other cases, the majority, this behaviour is different in nature, cannot be explained in terms of any known biological process, but is intelligible in terms of what concrete other persons in actual relationship to the patient do to him in interaction with him doing things to them. What we must do to avoid a fatal confusion is to distinguish between behaviour presenting in terms that are most appropriately seen as *explicable* process, and, on the other hand, behaviour that is *intelligible* in terms of what people are actually doing to each other. These differently presented problems imply a corresponding difference in method of approach. The fact that these totally different sorts of problem are contained within the same institution is one reason why the myth of disease process, with all its implicit violence, has been perpetuated in the case of schizophrenia. 'Schizophrenics', 'neurotics', 'psychopaths' have been placed in wards next to people with actual brain diseases. This dubious disease called 'schizophrenia' accounts for the great majority of mental hospital beds, and mental hospital beds constitute about half the hospital beds in this country.

In the popular mind the schizophrenic is the prototypical madman, he is the author of the totally gratuitous crazy act, the act that always has overtones of violence to others. He is the one who mocks the sane ones ('mannerism', 'grimacing', 'buffoonery', subtle forms of withdrawal), but at the same time concedes to them the ground for his own invalidation. He is the illogical man, the man whose logic is 'ill'. Or so they say. But perhaps we can discover some nuclear sense lying at the heart of this apparent nonsense. Where does he come from, this lunatic? Where does he come from and how does he get here in the midst of us? Is there just possibly a secret sanity concealed in this madness?

First, he is born into a family and this, some would say, is the highest common factor in his relation to the rest of us. But let us examine his family, assuming for the moment that this family is significantly different from most others.

In the family of the person destined to be designated schizo-phrenic we discover a peculiar sort of extremism. Even the most seemingly trivial issues are hinged around the polarities sanity/madness, life/death. The family group laws that regulate not only behaviour but also permissible experience are both confusing and inflexible. A child in such a family has to learn a mode of relating to, say, his mother upon which, he is taught, her very mental and physical integrity depends. He is taught that if he breaks the rules, and the most apparently innocuous autonomous act may constitute such a breach, he will cause both the fatal dissolution of the family group and the personal disintegration of his mother and possibly others. In this way, as R. D. Laing and A. Esterson (Laing, 1961; Laing and Esterson, 1964), have so clearly shown, he is progressively placed in an untenable position. His choice at the final critical point is only that between, on the one hand, total submission, the total abandonment of his freedom, and, on the other hand, departure from the group, which entails the anguish of witnessing the prophesied devastation of the others and contending with the guilt that has with such affectionate care been planted in him. Most destined schizophrenics find a synthetic answer to this dilemma which often coincides in the present state of affairs with that which their families find for them, namely to leave the family but to leave it to enter the mental hospital.

In the mental hospital, society has, with unerring skill, produced a social structure that in many respects reduplicates the madden-ing peculiarities of the patient's family. In the mental hospital he finds psychiatrists, administrators, nurses, who are his veritable parents, brothers, and sisters, who play an interpersonal game which only too often resembles in the intricacies of its rules the game he failed in at home. Once again he is perfectly free to choose. He may decide to vegetate his days away in a chronic back ward or he may decide to oscillate between his family hell and the not dissimilar hell of the conventional psychiatric admission ward – the latter course being the usual present-day idea of psychiatric progress. That is to say, schizophrenic patients may be discharged from hospital in less than three months, but about half of them are readmitted in less than a year. A course between these alternatives has yet to be discovered (see Appendix, p. 112).

But how does a person get into so unfortunate a position in which such violence is done to him? Basically, the situation is like this: mother and child form an original biological unit which persists some time after the physical fact of the child's birth. Then, bit by bit, the actions of the mother, if these are correct in a certain definable sense, engender a field of praxis with the possibility of reciprocity. There are two people who can do things with and to each other. The child then initiates action that affects the mother as the other to whom he is another. This beginning of action which affects another, or personal beginning, is the second birth or existential birth that dialectically transcends the original organismal reflex level and by attaining a new level of synthetic organization initiates a dialectic between persons. But the mother, for various reasons, may fail to generate on her side this field of reciprocal action, and it is in this sense that some people, in fact very many people, have never been born or, more usually, their birth has been only a shadow event and their lives represent only a marginal form of existence. Finally, even their death may be appropriated from them and become merely an event 'for others' – that is to say, the person lacks awareness of the direction of his life towards his personal death: he will never die *his* death since death for him is merely a statistical inevitability in the anonymous future. The job of a mother is to produce not only a child, but a field of possibilities in which her child may become someone else, another person.

So, the process of becoming a person may go wrong, and it may go wrong within the first few months of a life. If the mother fails to generate the field of reciprocal action so that the infant learns how to affect her as another, the child will lack the precondition for the realization of his personal autonomy. He will for ever be a thing, an appendage, something not quite human, a perfectly animated doll. This never happens absolutely but relatively to a widely varying degree it is common; in fact, a degree of failure is universal.

But the beginning of personal development is never a pure passivity. The acts of the mother are its precondition but never its cause. From the first moment of mother–child interaction, where each is another to the other, the child is in the position of having to initiate the project to become whoever he is to be, and this is, in principle, a free choice, his free creation of his essential nature.

For some people, however, not only is there a failure of the preconditional basis of their separate human existence, but once they have some precarious foothold on autonomy they are confused by others in their family with regard to the true nature of each intention they entertain and each act they perform. If such confusion is intensive and extensive enough, their position in the family may become untenable, and when this is the case violence is revealed quite naked.

Sometimes a person is fixed in the position where the only possible move he can make in the interpersonal game is one which is most likely to be termed 'violent' by *others*. Such is the case, for example, with the young man who has never been able to realize himself as a separate person from his mother. All the stratagems employed in the interest of love fail, because love demands reciprocation and there can be no real reciprocation in this case, since in the mother's view, and this view totally regulates the field, there can be no reciprocal field of action, no lover and no loved one. There is a perfect symbiosis where the symbiotic couple lose sight of the difference 'parasite/host' and become, almost in fact and certainly in phantasy, *one person*. For example, the fifty-year-old man in a chronic ward in the mental hospital who is dutifully taken home each weekend by his mother. She looks after him very well, of course. Like his ward charge nurse, she strips him, bathes him, inspects his body for signs of injury or disease, and then writes letters to his doctor expressing concern about the swelling on his left big toe which needs specialist attention. *She* usually gets it. In such a case the only move left to play seems to be that of apparently arbitrary, sudden, gratuitous, aggressive self-assertion on the part of the child. The child, who may be twenty, thirty, forty, or fifty years old is aggressive towards his mother as a means, the only means left, of breaking away from her. The rigorous logic of this situation is: 'If I hit you I am not you ... *I* am *me* since I hit *you* ... You are yourself since by hitting you I am another person ... You are another person ... you ... I am ... me.' Q.E.D.[1] In the clinical record a note is then made to the effect that his behaviour on this occasion was bizarre, irrational, and purposelessly violent.

It is only in the last ten years or so that some psychiatrists have begun to take into account the other side of the story of violence. It has been noted that the labelled schizophrenic patient is repeatedly confronted by contradictory demands in his family and sometimes in the psychiatric ward. This had been termed the 'double bind' by some American workers. I shall consider this notion in its theoretical context in the next chapter but can exemplify it here with the simple case where the mother makes a statement which she contradicts by gestures: She tells her son, 'Go away, find your own friends and don't be so dependent on me', but, at the same time, indicates non-verbally that she will be very upset if he does leave her, even in this limited way. Or, while signalling anxiety about any physical closeness, she says, 'Come and kiss your mother, dear!' Unless her child can discover a ruthlessness, a counter-violence, in himself with which he can demolish the whole absurd interchange, his response can only be muddle and ultimately what is called psychotic confusion, thought disorder, catatonia, and so on.

It is something like the situation expressed in certain Zen Buddhist koans where one is *fixed* in the position of having to make a response but each of the stated, alternative responses is predefined as wrong. This cannot be worked out rationally or analytically: the only answer must be an act that carries one from the false existential position in which one has been placed, a position in which one cannot exist, to a true self-centred rather

[1] This, needless to say, applies also to certain surrogate murders such as those done by Raskolnikov in *Crime and punishment*.

than other-centred position. But if one attempts to break out of the system of false rationality of the family, particularly when this system is reinforced by the collusion with the family of agents of the wider society, then one runs the risk of being called irrational. One might even have some 'disease' that has led to this madness. The fact that this irrationality is really a necessary anti-logic and not ill-logic and that the patient's violence is a necessary counter-violence may only too easily be overlooked. To a quite remarkable extent the 'illness' or the illogicality of the schizophrenic has its origin in the illness of the logic of other people.

So the family, then, in order to preserve itself in its inauthenic manner of living invents a disease. Medical science, sensitive to such widespread social needs, has provided a special discipline, psychiatry, to conceptualize, formalize, classify, and provide treatment for this disease.[1] The notion of disease-entity implies symptoms and the family prepares a formidable list of these. Schizophrenic symptoms are virtually whatever makes the family unbearably anxious about the tentatively independent behaviour of one of its offspring. These behavioural signs usually involve issues such as aggression, sexuality, and generally any form of autonomous self-assertion. These signs may well be the

---

[1] The medical establishment tends to regard psychiatry with condescension. This is only partly without justification. The justification resides in the fact that many psychiatrists have totally lost themselves in the intricacies of organic medicine, they take examinations in higher medicine, learn how to inspect the fundus of the eye and how to ascertain the exactly correct proportion of substances in our various excreta. They gradually and painstakingly acquire a requisite ignorance concerning the other person (patient) whom they confront or, more usually, refuse to confront. In fact, many psychiatrists are second-rate doctors – people who could not 'make it' in general medicine, but this fact does not limit the possibilities of pretence. The pretence breaks down, however, in certain cases – cases where the psychiatrist has actually tried to understand his patient on the basis of an understanding he has tried to achieve of himself – perhaps through lengthy and costly psycho-analytic training. This is a halting and imperfect course, perhaps, but one which the medical establishment and its hand-picked selection committees (for psychiatric jobs) show little sign of comprehending. For this reason, people who are humanly, technically, and professionally ill-equipped are thrust into positions of socio-medical power as consultants, superintendents, and even, sometimes, professors of psychiatry.

customary expression of the needs of an adolescent person, but, in certain families, even these are quite unacceptable and must, if necessary by some desperate means, be invalidated. A most respectable and readily available form of invalidation is to call such behaviour 'ill'. The ill patient is then removed from the family, with the co-operation of various social and medical agents, and the family is left to mobilize all its resources into pitying itself for the tragedy that has befallen it. Befallen it, of course, due to the hand of God which moves inexplicably and without relation to the actual needs of other people in the family.

I shall at this point refer to an actual case of this sort of thing. A patient was admitted to a mental hospital on a Detention Order (that is to say, a form of certification under the Mental Health Act of 1959 which removes from the patient his rights to leave hospital of his own accord, and if he does so provides for his forcible return to hospital by either police or hospital staff). The story was that this young man had, among other things which remained unspecified, behaved aggressively and violently towards his parents and that he, as the order stated, had to be removed for the protection of others to an institution for observation of his mental state. His parents had referred their problem to the general practitioner who, with the assistance of the Mental Welfare Officer, had issued the Detention Order. However, when one probed deeply enough into the circumstances of the family crisis one discovered that the aggressive and violent behaviour consisted in (a) breaking one tea-cup, (b) slamming the front door, and (c) stamping his foot once, but rather emphatically, on the garden path. In the course of the assessment of the family situation, which included a staged re-enactment of the 'crisis', it was discovered that the patient's mother had been struggling for many years with feelings of severe depression. At a certain moment in the history of the family when father, who was himself a depressed, totally withdrawn person, became crippled by a stroke, it became necessary for mother to rid herself of her intense feelings of guilt in order to cope with her new and difficult role of nurse, and the only person available for her as a receptacle for these feelings was her twenty-five-year-old son. Her son had, successfully enough, been conditioned to be such a receptacle. This situation, now at crisis point, had developed over three to four years. Her son, at the age of twenty-one, had had the usual feelings of extreme sensitivity about himself. He had projected unacceptable sexual and aggressive bits of himself into others and had experienced the return of these aspects of himself as ridicule and even persecution. This had led to an earlier admission to hospital in which he had proclaimed the delusional idea that he was Jesus Christ. At that time, as on the present occasion, he was bearing vicariously the full load of his mother's guilt, and in the micro-social family world he was dying in order that the others, principally his mother, might be saved. We all repeatedly die partial deaths in order that the others, for whom we are the sacrificial offerings, may live. The archetypal Christ, in so far as he has any reality at all, is in each of us. In this sense the patient's delusional proclamation was quite true, but it was a truth that no one else could allow himself to see. If one reads the score this way, one appreciates the dictum of the American psychiatrist who defined delusion as a true idea held by the patient which the psychiatrist deludes himself into accepting literally. But the opposite of the literal is not necessarily the metaphorical. The existential reality of a person transcends this opposition.

When this young man comes into the mental observation ward we find that these obvious facts are either excluded from consideration or that they are distorted in a uniformly peculiar way, and if we are to understand the reality of psychiatric violence we shall have to get some idea of what the distortion is.

The mental patient, once he has been so labelled, is obliged to take a sick role. Essential to this role is a certain passivity. There is supposed to be a disease which, coming somehow from outside the person, is a process that alters him. The patient is affected, altered in such a manner that his own affecting and altering become relatively inessential. He is reified to become the object in which the disease-process works itself out. The process is suffered, undergone. No one, it is supposed, does anything at all until the *mise en scène* of the psychiatrist who (sometimes, and usually disastrously) cures the rot. The disease happens to the person who, in so far as this is a mere happening, becomes quite literally no one at all. As the bearer of symptoms that result from a process, he is dispensable as a person and, therefore, is dispensed with. One is left with the doctor who confronts an inert non-human field of symptoms (which must always be removed or suppressed) and disease process (which must, if possible, be eliminated). This pre-structuring of the situation that arises when someone enters the mental hospital immediately implies that what has gone on between the elected patient and other persons has a significance (if it has any at all) that is only secondary to the supposed disease. To say this by no means implies malevolence or even a lack of 'human warmth' in the doctor.

The recognition of such violence finds its closest parallel in current psychiatric thinking in the concept of 'institutionalization' in the mental hospital. But it is ironic that this critique of institutionalization has itself fallen into the trap of institutionalized thinking, in particular when it produces ideas such as that of 'institutional neurosis'. The invention of this curious disease (yet another disease) has led one of its protagonists to list causal factors, symptoms, diagnosis, prognosis, and treatment. If one cannot find a real virus, one invents a social virus.

On the ground that it does violence to human reality, we must question this whole way of thinking, centred on the notion of passivity, of being altered by a disease process, biological and/or psychological and/or social.

This disease (or diseased) way of thinking, however, is firmly rooted in the medical tradition in which the work that psychiatrists do, for certain historical reasons, has become enmeshed. But whereas the disease idea functions reasonably and serviceably in general medicine and its other specialities, its wholesale transplantation into a field where problems are presented in terms of relationships between persons has produced confusion and formidable contradictions on every level of theory and meta-theory—although the latter level is rarely attained and never sustained in the clinical psychiatric literature, for the very reason that one cannot make a theoretical study, within a continuous framework of reference, of a theory which is self-contradictory in its most basic elements. The most advanced and radical critique of psychiatric theory in terms of its false conceptual model must propose an analysis of psychiatry and psycho-analysis in their historical origins.[1]

In concrete fact, there is very little explicit awareness about what is really happening when someone goes into a mental hospital ward. Not only does the patient's physical bed await him in the ward, but there is also a Procrustean bed of staff preconceptions into which he must be fitted at whatever cost in terms of mutilation of his personal reality. The violence that commences in his family is perpetuated in the conventional psychiatric ward. Most apparent psychiatric progress expressed in the catchwords 'open doors', 'permissiveness', 'informality', 'friendly staff-patient relations', serves to obscure this far more central area in which the traditional psychiatric hospital has not advanced one inch since the days of Kraepelin in the last century.

It is a truism to say that the patient's relationships with his family, his doctor, and other significant persons must be taken into consideration when we have to decide how best to act in relation to him to be 'therapeutic'. Of course, this is done, at least in principle, in all but the most backward psychiatric institutions. It is, however, still almost revolutionary to suggest that the problem lies not in the so-called 'ill person' but in the interacting network of persons, particularly his family, from which the admitted patient, by a piece of conceptual sleight of hand, has already been abstracted. Madness, that is to say, is not 'in' a

[1] See Szasz, T. S. (1962). Szasz deals paradigmatically almost exclusively with hysteria, showing what violence is done to the existence of the hysterical person by construing the main aspects of his behaviour as symptoms of a mysterious disease process; but while his examination of this pseudo-disease amply supports his thesis, I believe that a similarly orientated examination of the whole field of psychiatric madness does so even more strongly.

28

person, but in a system of relationships in which the labelled 'patient' participates: schizophrenia, if it means anything, is a more or less characteristic mode of disturbed group behaviour. There are no schizophrenics. The usual abstraction of an 'ill person' from the system of relationships in which he is caught up immediately distorts the problem and opens the way to the invention of pseudo-problems which are then quite seriously classified and analysed causally – all genuine problems having vanished unnoticed through the hospital gates (along with the departing relatives).

Attributions of strangeness, queerness, oddity, craziness, incongruity or absence of feelings, purposeless acts, impulsiveness or unreasoning aggression, are not unquestionable, absolute, or even (in ordinary clinical experience) reasonably objective judgements about the patient-to-be when they are made by other members of his family. These attributions are highly functional and they function in relation to a system of needs in the family at a certain point in its history. Nor are attributions of madness made by agents of the extra-familial society, in particular general practitioner and Mental Welfare Officer, occasionally the police, necessarily more objective than those made by the family. Only too often they fall into a rather subtle, skilfully (albeit unconsciously) prepared collusion with the family attitudes.

This collusive relation between family and the agents of society is the basis of real as opposed to mythical violence in psychiatry. It has not been nor will it remain an eternal characteristic of the social system. In mediaeval times the present boundaries between family and extra-familial community did not exist. Not only was the family 'out' in the community far more than it is today, but also the household, especially in the case of the upper classes, included many extra-familial others – servants, nurse-maids, guests. As soon as the child emerged from early infantile dependence he became, in the eyes of the adults, as the iconography of the period confirms, a 'miniature adult'. In the sixteenth, seventeenth, and particularly the eighteenth century the situation began to change: the *rites de passage* which from neolithic times had initiated the child into his adult identity (often through symbolic death, or the partial death of symbolic castration and reversal of sexual identity, and the conferring of a new name), these and the Hellenistic *paideia* had all disappeared in mediaeval Europe; in the eighteenth century a preoccupation with the nature of childhood and the transition into adult life reappeared.[1]

Henceforth it was recognized that the child as a special sort of person, a special, rather disturbing presence, should have a special preparation, and education, for his adult role in life. The child was segregated from the life of the adult community by family and school, often in a harshly monastic manner in the claustrating total institution of the boarding-school. The attendant brutalities, however, reflected not the mediaeval indifference to the child as a child but an obsessive, imprisoning family love. Here indeed we see love as violence.

The widely proclaimed contemporary evidence for the loosening of family bonds (e.g. the divorce rate and weakening of paternal authority) does little but transparently mask a peculiar sort of intensification of family cohesion in our society – a cohesion for which we may discover the historical intelligibility. The concept of 'a family', which differs significantly from the demographic institution, implies a family-community boundary-line and is a phenomenon of modern history; before the sixteenth to eighteenth century, class divisions, although always objectively definable, were often blurred in the actual processes of social intercourse and the denumerable members of each family were all very much part of the total community; after the eighteenth century the early development of the basic contradictions of capitalist society limited the blurring of class distinctions, which became less tolerable to the upper classes, who began to withdraw socially, geographically (to special districts), and in terms of the upbringing of children. Henceforth values of privacy, the immuration of the family, reigned – to some extent imitatively reproduced in working-class life in so far as this was con-

[1] This thesis is expounded and amply documented by Philippe Ariès (1960) in 'Centuries of childhood'.

ditioned by the values imposed by the ruling upper and middle classes.

We can think this out in terms of the categories suggested by Claude Lévi-Strauss in *Tristes Tropiques* (1955). There are societies which swallow people up, namely anthropophagic societies, and societies which vomit people out – anthropoemic societies. We then see a transition from, on the one hand, the mediaeval 'swallowing up' of the child-person in the community, a mode of assimilative acceptance relating to ritualistic cannibalism in 'primitive' societies in which the ritual enabled people to accept the unacceptable – particularly death – to, on the other hand, the anthropoemic modern society which ejects from itself all that it cannot draw into accepting the artfully invented rules of its game. On this basis it excludes facts, theories, attitudes, and people – people of the wrong class, the wrong race, the wrong school, the wrong family, the wrong sexuality, the wrong mentality. In the traditional psychiatric hospital today, despite the proclamation of progress, society gets the best of both worlds – the person who is 'vomited' out of his family, out of society, is 'swallowed up' by the hospital and then digested and metabolized out of existence as an identifiable person. This, I think, must be regarded as violence.

The process of getting rid of someone is, of course, denied, usually by some form of assertion of the inherent peculiar badness and madness of certain individuals. This denial, which operates both in the family and in the wider society, is that most sterile, tortuous and yet all-pervasive piece of social illogic, the negation of the negation. The steps of the process are as follows: First, there is a negative act, an act of invalidation of a person by others; this may involve diagnostic labelling, passing sentence, physically removing the person from his social context: second (concurrently, rather than chronologically after), this negative act is denied in various ways; it is held that the person has invalidated himself or has been invalidated by his inherent weaknesses or disease process, other persons have nothing much to do with the matter. By means of this double negation the social group conceals its praxis from itself. The 'good', 'sane' people, who define themselves as such by defining certain of their number as 'mad' and 'bad' and then extruding them from the group, maintain a safe and comfortable homeostasis by this lie about a lie. The elected scapegoats often collude with this process, often finding that the only way they can feel needed by others or confirmed in a definite enough identity is by taking a mad or bad social role. The 'delusion' of being Christ, of sacrificing oneself for the sake of humanity, as we saw in the earlier example, finds its intelligibility in terms of this inauthentic social praxis.

When society is a little less dishonest about what it is up to one discovers analogous forms of practice expressed much more obviously and concretely. In illustrating his thesis that all social evil is projection, Sartre in his book on Jean Genet (1952, p. 29), describes an industry which once flourished in Bohemia. The 'normal' adults took little children, split their lips, compressed their skulls and imprisoned them day and night in boxes to prevent growth. By this means they were able to produce 'monsters' which could be publicly exhibited at a profit. Today, in the case of labelled lunatics, society is developing a rudimentary awareness of guilt in connection with the production and maintenance of a segregated mad sub-community. This guilt is manifested in contradictory efforts to improve the status of mental patients by promoting them to the rank of ordinary sick people, and by greater permissiveness in psychiatric institutions, but, on the other hand, to keep them in their mad role by the whole pseudo-medical system of patient identification and confirmation and by a host of difficulties of obscure origin in the rehabilitation process. In the setting of this quasi-medical mystique the periodic bursts of frenetic therapeutic activity directed by some psychiatrists against their schizophrenic patients does little but perpetuate the irrationality of the system.

Antonin Artaud, the eminent writer and theorist of the 'theatre of cruelty', has written some very relevant things about this. There were long dialogues between Artaud and his psychiatrists in which Artaud defended his belief that he was the victim of voodoo spells and defended his right to withdraw from other people. In opposition to this, the psychiatrist would painstakingly spell out the need for him to conform with society. And so it would go on. But at the final critical moment of the dialogue the rub was always this: 'If you speak of bewitchment again, M. Artaud, you shall have 65 electro-shocks.' There is a sense in which Artaud's 'delusional statements' represented a profound reality in life, a reality which, seventeen years after his death, we are only just beginning to appreciate; he had more to say relevant to madness than all the textbooks of psychiatry, but the trouble was that Artaud saw too much and spoke too much of the truth. He had to be cured. It is perhaps not too absurd to say that it is very often when people start to become *sane* that they enter the mental hospital.

If we are to advance from the present position in psychiatry where the violence of which I have been speaking is so widely prevalent, we shall have to recognize the dialectical complexity of human reality and refuse to reduce all human action and experience to process terms. We shall have to seek the vital moment of praxis, the intentional core of each human existence, the project by which each person defines himself in the world. This has always been difficult to accomplish in the large traditional psychiatric institution and, in practical terms, our experience suggests that what is needed is a small community of about thirty or forty people which will function without the usual clinical preconceptions and prejudices, without rigid, externally imposed staff–patient hierarchization, and with full and active involvement of families of people in the community. In such an 'experimental' community a person will not have to contend with the alienated desires of others who try to beat him into shape, to cure him of trying to become the person he really is. He will at last have the chance to discover and explore authentic relatedness to others. Such a community does not yet exist but may be created.

In the meantime, if one has to go mad, the tactic to learn in our society is one of discretion.

33

CHAPTER II

Families and Schizophrenia

The strategists have a saying,
I dare not play the host but play the guest,
I dare not advance an inch but retreat a foot instead.
This is known as marching forward when there is no road,
Rolling up one's sleeves when one has no arm,
Dragging one's adversary by force when there is no adversary,
And taking up arms when there are no arms.
Lao Tzu, *Tao Te Ching*, Book II, LXIX

To a query of Mang Wu respecting filial piety, the Master replied: 'Parents ought to bear but one trouble — that of their own sickness.'
The Confucian Analects, Book II, 6

Since the earliest days of institutional psychiatry, nurses, and sometimes psychiatrists, have had shrewd intuitions that, however disturbed the admitted schizophrenic patient seemed to be, he was not alone in his disturbance. Quite often experienced staff have guessed that something unusual, or even crazy, has been going on in the family of the patient, and this feeling has been expressed in remarks such as 'perhaps we've got the wrong one in here'.

The usual mental hospital procedure with regard to the patient's relatives has been that they are interviewed by the psychiatrist, perhaps on one occasion only and without the presence of the patient. At some hospitals, routine inquiry forms about the patient's past life and 'present illness' are posted to the next of kin without the patient's knowledge. Occasionally, a psychiatric social worker, at some stage of the patient's career as a patient,

34

has an opportunity to see him together with his family at home, but this is by no means the rule and, in most instances, is limited to a traditional type of casework that does not comprehend the more recent insights into the workings of families with which I shall deal in this chapter. These new insights challenge very deeply traditional ideas that family environmental factors affect only superficial aspects of the 'illness' in the patient, or that the family is only secondarily affected by the 'pathology' of the patient.

First we must try to ascertain what a family is and what it does.

Many sociologists after Talcott Parsons have considered the family functionally in terms of, first, the primary socialization of the infant by the family and, secondly, the processes of stabilization of the adolescent and adult personality. If the family and its child members are not to be considered 'deviant' this biphasic indoctrination in the micro-culture (the family) must succeed in instilling the values and behavioural norms of the macro-culture (the extra-familial world). In a society in which self-alienation is the rule, these values will be alienated values. The male child will be taught to regard himself and the skills he acquires as objects in the market, he will be provided with a framework in which he will identify positively and negatively (in suitable proportions) with his father, whose duty it is to *represent* his adequate self-esteeming and other-esteemed social role in the family circle. It is definitive of the conformist society that the parent's *representation* of an acceptable social role has priority over his *presentation* of himself to the child. The parent externalizes himself in the world, he empties his subjective reality into an object form of being-in-the-world, and then re-internalizes this objectification. But this presence that he re-internalizes is something he has already lost, it is, in fact, an *absence* that he represents in the family. The existential structure of the represented social role is that it is, first of all, being-for-the-other and then, secondly, it is being-for-oneself. Fortunately, not all families manage to escape entirely the stigma of deviance.

What we must really try to grasp is the notion of *autonomy* of each member of the family in the family. Autonomy means, first, laying down the law for oneself, self-rule, and this implies an act of rupture by which a person breaks and breaks out of an imprisoning system in which his role, like that of each other's, is only that of embodying the projections of another and then vicariously living out these vague hopes, ambitions, gratifying or punishing internalized traces of his parents, and so on. What he has to do to break out is most simply and yet very complexly to accept into himself this crazy mass of primitive relatedness, to bear this disturbing interiorization right up to the limit of its intrusion into him, and then to surpass it towards his own field of possibilities. In doing this he has to maintain his self-centredness, his existing himself from the subjective centre of his being outwards into the world. Should he lose his grasp on the centre of himself he loses himself to others and this means losing himself to himself, or rather from himself.

Alienation, then, refers to action and to the act of denial of action in a group and to the results of this action. Estrangement we shall understand as the experience of this result of alienated action. Estrangement is the feeling of being caught up in a process which is alien to one's own intentions and acts and to the intentions and acts of each other in the group. It is the experiential by-product of a universal illusion.

Families mediate social reality to their children. If the social reality in question is rife with alienated social forms, then this alienation will be mediated to the individual child and will be experienced as estrangement in the family relationships. Some of the 'closest' families and the 'happiest' marriages are those in which relations are most estranged. Estrangement may be evaded and denied. One may become estranged from one's estrangement. But if, for reasons that we can make intelligible, this denial becomes impossible, then a person may attempt to lessen his painful confusion by making a 'psychotic' construction – for example, he may say that his mind is controlled by an electrical machine or by men from outer space. These constructions, however, are largely embodiments of the family process, which

36

has the illusion of substantiality but which is nothing other than the alienated form of the action or praxis of the family members that literally dominates the mind of the psychotic member. These metaphorical men from outer space are the literal mother, father, and sibling who sit around the breakfast table with the so-called psychotic patient. In everyday discourse we habitually confuse the literal and the metaphorical. Who is to say that in this instance the patient is mad because he is metaphorical?

What I have been saying about alienated family relationships is very well brought out in Ionesco's play *The bald prima donna* (1950). A man and woman meet apparently as total strangers. They gradually discover that they have shared a train compartment, a house, a bed, a child. They conclude in amazement that they are one and the same family. Here relationship is defined by a tracing of non-human topographical relations – railroad, stairs, bed. But then how many husbands and wives *have* met each other – even remotely.

Families of psychiatric patients who are called schizophrenic exhibit this sort of alienation and estrangement in a particularly intense form. There is a very real sense in which the schizophrenia problem and the problem of alienation and estrangement in families are identical. It might be objected that we must await the results of controlled comparative investigation of families who have an identified psychotic member, or a neurotic member, and families none of whose members are diagnosed as ill in the psychiatric sense. My own work with families, however, has led me to suspect that both 'psychotic' and 'neurotic' families and 'normal' families are, in our community, characterized by a high degree of alienation from the personal reality of each of their members. One is even tempted to ponder on the daring hypothesis that in the 'psychotic' families the identified schizophrenic patient member by his psychotic episode is trying to break free of an alienated system and is, therefore, in some sense less 'ill' or at least less alienated than the 'normal' offspring of the 'normal' families. In so far as he enters a mental hospital, however, his

37

desperate attempt to liberate himself would seem to fail in terms of his deficiency in the necessary social tactics and strategy.

I have already introduced the term 'alienation' but if we are to extend our understanding of violence, we should now explore further its meaning. As a philosophical term 'alienation' was first used at the beginning of the nineteenth century by Fichte and Hegel. In the 1840s it was employed in the analysis of society by Marx. For most people, however, the notion of alienation in Marx's early work was overshadowed by certain aspects of his later theory and it had to await resuscitation in the last few decades of this century.

Hegel's original notion of alienation (*Entfremdung*) was rooted in his analysis of consciousness. In the work of some of his followers it took on the meaning of a condition in which human powers appeared in an externalized form as autonomous non-human entities, dominating human life 'from the outside'. In Feuerbach's analysis of religion, for example, gods and devils were seen as projections of aspects of human nature. From this base-line Marx extended the idea of alienation to cover many other forms of social life. The State was seen by Marx not as an autonomous external power dominating men, but as an alienated form of human action, namely the concerted praxis whereby one class of men dominated another class. The State in this sense is what is 'stated', posited, set up by those who are its liege subjects.

Sartre (1960) has sought the ontological basis of alienation. He regarded Marx's account of alienation in terms of exploitation and its social products as secondary alienation. Primary alienation, which is a necessary form of all human action and experience, consists in the categories of 'alteration', whereby 'my acts for myself' become 'my acts for the other', and of 'objectification', whereby my acts become actually and recordably impressed on the physical or social reality of the world. Sartre develops his earlier ideas (1943) of existential haemorrhage. That is to say, when I am regarded by another person there is an outward movement, 'bleeding', from my inner state of being-for-myself to an outer state of my being-for-the-other as an object in the world. This involves an interplay between two sorts of space. The sort of space 'I' occupy in being-for-myself is very different from that which the 'me' as an object for the other occupies. The eyes of the other as he looks at me may be, say, two yards away, but his *look* is right inside me, it penetrates the space of my subjectivity and would make me wholly an object for him. There is no measurable distance involved. Usually this outflowing of myself is checked by my reciprocal objectification of the other so that his existence, in turn under my regard, bleeds into the world of objects for me.

Some people suffer a continual invasion of their subjective space by others, so much so that finally their existence seems to become only that of an object in the geometrical systems of need of other members of the group. One has no space of one's own. In fact, it takes a great deal of deciding to go on living in such a way, but all the appearances are that such a person never does anything, he is wholly the summated effect of group (and possibly organismal) processes which obscure everything that he really does (his praxis), and therefore everything he is. He is totally alienated, but it is always a *person* who is alienated and this person is alienated through his continuously operating consenting intentionality. None the less, we should now see clearly the link between alienation and the violence that goes on in families.

Alienation in this sense is the source of numerous mythologies in social and psychological thinking in which there is the explicit or implicit positing of the human group as a sort of hyperorganism to which is attributed the capacity to act and even experience somehow independently of its members. This hyperorganism appears to follow its own independent laws. The obvious advantage of this way of thinking is that it provides an illusory exit from personal responsibility. In fact, the laws of the group are made in and through the interaction of each with each other and have their origin in the freedom of each member, in the freely chosen servitude to or rejection of already established group rules by each group member. Alienation as an exit from the disturbance and anguish of recognizing personal responsibility provided Eichmann with his 'defence' in terms of his being only 'a cog in the wheel'.

On the other hand, there is the story related by Bruno Bettelheim in *The informed heart* (1961) about a girl who, in an extreme moment of insight, recognized and broke out of one of the most formidable pieces of alienation in all human history. This girl was one of a group of Jews queueing naked to enter the gas chamber. The S.S. officer supervising proceedings heard that she had been a ballet dancer and ordered her to dance. She danced, but gradually approached the officer and suddenly seized his revolver and shot him. Her fate was obvious and it was equally obvious that nothing she could do could alter the physical facts of the situation, namely the extermination of the group. But what she did was to invest her death with an intense personal meaning that at the same time expressed an historic opportunity that was tragically lost in the massified process of the extermination camps.

Systematic research into the families of schizophrenic patients may, for practical purposes, be regarded as having commenced fifteen years ago in the United States, and this is a point we should reflect on. The psychiatrist Kraepelin in 1896 first grouped together various 'clinical pictures' under the name earlier suggested by C. Morel, 'dementia praecox' (later to be termed by Bleuler 'schizophrenia'). Since that time a great deal of research has been carried out into the bowel habits, thyroid function, etc., of schizophrenic patients. One savant demonstrated, or thought he had demonstrated, statistically that most schizophrenic patients were born in the month of March and produced a series of hypotheses to account for this 'fact'. Psychiatrists have divided and subdivided the 'clinical pictures' into thirty to forty different types and sub-types, using all the resources of Greek etymology they could muster for this labelling marathon. It may well seem a little strange to the unprejudiced outsider that no one thought it worth while, until fifteen years ago, to have a really close look at what went on in the families from which the patients were admitted. Or rather, it may seem strange until one considers the curious collusion which doctors and other agents of society have traditionally operated with the other members of the patient's family – usually his parents.

The first studies in 1949 and the early 1950s centred on the nature of the relationship between the parents of the schizophrenic patient and showed that in a very high proportion of cases this relationship was grossly unsatisfactory according to various criteria. Some of these early studies attempted to describe the predominant traits of the family members: the mother of the patient was usually regarded as an emotionally manipulative, dominating, over-protective and yet at the same time rejecting person, while the father was seen as characteristically weak, passive, preoccupied, ill, or, in some other sense, 'absent' as an effective person in the family.

In 1958 M. Bowen described what he called 'emotional divorce' between the parents in these families and it was clear that this sort of split might not be immediately obvious. In the same year L. C. Wynne *et al.* used the term 'pseudo-mutuality' to account for the manner in which some families present the appearance of mutuality and concord but only to cover over intense hostility, inflexibility, and mutual destructiveness. Wynne, in this work, has extended sociological role theory in a most pertinent and useful way by taking more account than is usual of the subjective experience of the role-taker. He and his co-workers consider complementarity in families in terms of mutual, non-mutual, and pseudo-mutual complementarity. In the case of mutuality there is greater differentiation and flexibility in family relatedness, which allows a deepening of relationship (which Wynne conceptualizes in Buberian terms). In non-mutuality there is a general lack of interest in the family in dealing with any perceptions of non-complementarity. In the families of certain schizophrenics, however, there is pseudo-mutuality which, it is hypothesized, takes on an especially enduring and intense form in these families and is reinforced by a family subculture of myths and idiosyncratic ideology of unusual pervasiveness, with dire mythical retribution awaiting the family member who dares cease to conform with this system. Wynne indicates, but only in outline, how the interiorization of this family system of relations conditions the development of the personal experience of each member.

A decisive new development in thinking out family interaction was brought about in 1956 by Gregory Bateson, Don Jackson, J. Haley, and J. H. Weakland, working at Palo Alto, California, in their paper 'Toward a theory of schizophrenia'. In this paper they elaborated the idea of a 'double-bind' manœuvre in families of schizophrenics as a factor contributing to the genesis of schizophrenia in one elected member. Weakland (1960) has summarized what is meant by a double-bind:

'The general characteristics of this (double-bind) situation are the following:

1. When the individual is involved in an intense relationship; that is, a relationship in which he feels it is vitally important that he discriminate accurately what sort of message is being communicated so that he may respond appropriately.

2. And, the individual is caught in a situation in which the other person in the relationship is expressing two orders of message and one of these denies the other.

3. And, the individual is unable to comment on the messages being expressed to correct his discrimination of what order of message to respond to, i.e. he cannot make a metacommunicative statement.'

So impossible is the dilemma of the schizophrenic or schizophrenic-to-be when he is presented with this manœuvre by one or both of his parents that the only response he can make is one that is conventionally regarded as psychotic. But in the social reality of the family in which he lives and in which he has grown up he has internalized a peculiar restriction of his field of possibilities by virtue of which these psychotic responses may be the most reasonable reactions possible until the social field changes, either through a change in the family, which may be provoked by an external intervention, or by the removal of the identified patient to a social group where metacommunicative awareness is part of the group currency. This latter group may be either an ideologically advanced therapeutic group or any other relatively non-mystifying group of people.

A fairly common example of double-binding occurs frequently in conjoint family interviews in which the patient meets together with his parents, and possibly siblings, and the therapist. Here the patient is enjoined by one of his parents to recall some incident in the family history which is relevant to the issue under discussion but which is clearly laden with emotions that are threatening to the rest of the family or to one of its members. Simultaneously with this injunction to remember, the enjoiner emits a paralinguistic or entirely non-verbal injunction (for example, signs, visible to the patient, of great anxiety) to the effect that if he dare recall and state the relevant point he will dangerously menace or even destroy the family or at least one of its members. At the same time there are contextually built-in injunctions neither to comment on the secondary non-verbal injunction nor to evade the question. The patient then responds with some 'thought-disordered' statement expressing inability to use his mind properly and remember some obviously significant and perhaps fairly recent happening. He both experiences confusion and expresses muddle.

The importance of this work resides in the fact that the authors have finally got on to a microscopic analysis of each statement and even each non-verbal nuance in the family interaction. They have also indicated how the patient, by interiorizing these contradictory signal systems, may both inwardly experience confusion and then exteriorize this confusion by objectifying himself, in the family group and its social periphery which includes the psychiatric interview situation, as 'a muddled person' or 'a schizophrenic' in one important sense of this term.

In their further theoretical development, however, these authors seem to me to fall short of an adequate conceptualization of the underlying processes. They resort to Bertrand Russell's

43

notion of 'logical types'[1] as this was originally formulated in *Principia mathematica* (1913). They hold that the two contradictory messages presented to the patient are of different logical types, but that the patient has been conditioned not to perceive this difference and is therefore subject to logical-type confusion and is therefore a ready victim to the double-bind. This seems to me to be an *ad hoc* conjunction of concepts which adds nothing to the authors' most lucid description of the double-bind situation as it is experienced. The point, as far as logic is concerned, is that the double-binding party implicitly proposes a false logical model to the doubly-bound party – in short an analytic rationality appropriate to physical and biological action-reaction systems but not to personal interaction. Personal interaction, particularly in so far as one makes logical inferences regarding it, must be seen dialectically. The anthropological logician in his logical system must observe that the objects of the system are bivalent in the sense that the double-binder simultaneously wants and does not want, or rather needs and does not need, a certain response from the other. The need of the parents in our example for their child to remember the fateful event is a real, socially conditioned need and not a pure 'phoney'. But it runs counter to another socially conditioned need – for the child to forget. The truth of the matter is that the double-binders are, in fact, the ones who are doubly-bound by the convergence of contradictory social forces on them: first, needs conditioned by the general social field of expectations in which they have been brought up and, secondly, needs to preserve the family (of procreation) structure such as it is in the face of a threat presented by the patient member who would dare assert himself autonomously. The parents, however, deny the contradictory moment of their own situation and believe that when they ask 'do you remember?', they are asking a single, simple unambiguous question (although there is certainly also, in many

[1] In brief, if one takes a proposition p and then asserts a proposition p^1 about proposition p, in which p is one term of the proposition p^1, then proposition p is of the first logical type and p^1 is of the second logical type. Similarly, proposition p^2, which is about p^1, is of the third logical type.

cases, some conscious duplicity). Furthermore, invoking conventional family rights and obligations, they insist on a simple, unambiguous answer. In doing so they clearly demand the moon.

The real illogic, or illness of logic, is then seen to be in the parents in so far as they resort to an inappropriate type of rationality (which subsumes Russell's logical typology) to defend their position. The truth is, however, that society in general errs in this way whenever it speaks either of intimate personal relations or of its own large-scale historical development. This can be seen in the types of statement made about human motivation in courts of law and also in massified political judgements. The defensive shift from dialectical to analytical rationality is brought about whenever an individual or group threatens to assert himself or itself autonomously. The omnipresent threat is the independent breakaway – whatever form it takes.

If one states the schizophrenia problem this way, namely in terms of the existence of a person being sucked out of him by others, or expressed from him by himself (in loving acknowledgement of the others' rapacious ingestion) so that finally nothing of himself is left to himself since he is altogether for the other, then we must conclude that, although being put in hospital represents a special fate, schizophrenia is nothing less than the predicament of each one of us.

CHAPTER III

Studying One Family

'And a woman who held a babe against her bosom said, 'Speak to us of Children.'

And he said:

'Your children are not your children.

They are the sons and daughters of Life's longing for itself.

They come through you but not from you,

And though they are with you yet they belong not to you.

You may give them your love but not your thoughts,

For they have their own thoughts.

You may house their bodies but not their souls,

For their souls dwell in the house of to-morrow, which you cannot visit, not even in your dreams.

You may strive to be like them, but seek not to make them like you.

For life goes not backward nor tarries with yesterday.

You are the bows from which your children as living arrows are sent forth.

The archer sees the mark upon the path of the infinite, and He bends you with His might that His arrows may go swift and far.

Let your bending in the Archer's hand be for gladness;

For even as He loves the arrow that flies, so He loves also the bow that is stable.'

Kahlil Gibran, *The Prophet*

'Schizophrenia is caused by the fact that young people no longer obey their parents.'

Journal of Mental Science (1904, p. 272)

In each case the problem is to take the behaviour of the identified schizophrenic patient and attempt to discover to what extent this

46

behaviour is intelligible in terms of the interaction between this
person and other persons in the past and in the present.

In the cases we have studied[1] 'behaviour' includes most specifically the so-called 'clinical presentation of the illness' on and just
prior to admission to hospital – the 'presenting psychotic symptoms'.
'Other persons' for our present purposes means the patient's nuclear
family (his mother, father, and siblings), in some cases marital
partner, and also staff and other patients in the ward community.

The 'material' for analysis is collected by participant-observers,
first in group situations with the families. Participant-observation
means that the observer participates in a group interaction and that
he is aware of and records his mode of participation and its effect
in the total interaction as an essential part of the observational
procedure. Participation is both an inevitable and an intrinsic part
of this situation. Also in most of the interactions we have recorded
there has been the clear intention to carry out 'family therapy'.
Therapeutic interventions in this sense do not aim primarily at the
interpretation of unconscious phantasy but assume the form of
meta-communications (communications about communications)
aimed at clarifying confusions that may be introduced by the
primary communications – many of which are already communications about communications. Although we state that
interpretation of unconscious phantasy is not our primary aim, it
often happens that a meta-communicative intervention brings
into group awareness 'unconscious processes'.

Second, participant-observations are made in the ward groups
which include the patient during his stay in hospital. The
'therapeutic' organizing principles of these groups, which help to
define the nature of the observations, are described in Chapter IV.

Family interactions selected for study are tape-recorded, and
the recordings are transcribed into typescript. Non-verbal
communications, however, unless cinematographic techniques
are used, have to be noted as they occur by the observer in the
group. Some of the para-linguistic aspects – intonation, inflection
of voice, etc. – come through on the tape-recording.

[1] In my unit described in the following two chapters.

47

The patient is usually first seen in an interview on his admission to the unit. This is the procedure in all 'urgent' admissions from home, but in some cases, when for example the patient is referred for admission from an out-patient clinic, the whole family, or perhaps the patient and one parent, are seen together on the first encounter and invited to state the problem, perhaps in the form 'Could someone say what the trouble seems to be?' After a two-person interview with a doctor, the patient entering the unit becomes part of the ward community group and in the earlier phases of the unit's functioning he would a little later be invited to join a group engaged in one of the work projects: to some extent he would choose his work group, but there were naturally limits to the maximum or minimum number of people who could work on a certain project. He is also expected to do his share of ward domestic work (cleaning, laying the dining-tables, and washing up). Finally he will participate in the various organized and informal social and recreational groups, usually with staff present.

The family investigation is a part of the total investigation, which in a given case may take anything from three to four hours up to forty to fifty hours of investigation and therapeutic time. On the basis of an initial family assessment, plus assessment of the patient's problems as evident in the ward group interactions, the amount of time to be spent with the family is decided by the doctor therapist. It is decided in fact whether a number of sessions of family therapy are indicated; therapy, that is to say, in the sense of an attempt to modify the existing patterns of interaction in the family or, rather, therapy as *the provision of a controlled situation in which the family members modify themselves in relation to each other in such a way that the identified patient member discovers an increasing area of autonomous action for himself, while at the same time the other family members become more 'self-sufficient', at least to the extent of not breaking down in a manner judged to be psychotic.*

In certain cases (the majority, partly due to limitations of therapist time) it may be decided not to involve the whole family to any extent directly in the therapeutic situation; then the aim of work with the patient will be more simply to provide the sort of situation in which he will find social experiences, transitional from his family experience, which lead to his being able to exist in the community without becoming the focus of attributions of mental illness. If this works out well, he learns to exist independently of his family and ultimately of the ward. Often he graduates through the stages of full 'in-patient' status, then working out from the ward in a local job, then living in lodgings and attending only once a week or fortnight for an out-patient session. In other cases, on the basis of the initial family assessment, it may be decided that some other member of the family who more or less willingly takes the role of primary patient may come into an inpatient or outpatient therapeutic situation and the original patient admitted with schizophrenia may be promptly discharged: in our experience in the unit this sick-role reversal has happened most often between 'normal' mothers and 'schizophrenic' sons.

The admitted patient is interviewed alone for at least one hour-long session by the doctor. The whole family, at least the parents and the patient, siblings too if available, meet with the doctor for a variable number of hour-long sessions. Various dyads and triads from the family meet in similar sessions, the main combinations, in addition to the basic whole family group, being the two parents together, each parent in turn with the schizophrenic child, and a 'non-schizophrenic' sibling together with the patient. There are also two-persons sessions in which each parent in turn and at least one sibling see the doctor alone. These latter sessions are particularly apt to bring out highly contradictory views of the patient, his 'illness', and the family (Laing and Esterson, 1964).

There are two interview rooms in which the families may meet. In one they sit around a table, in the other there is a circle of armchairs. Consent for tape-recording the sessions is obtained before the machine is switched on – we have never experienced any objection to tape-recording or undue conscious preoccupation with the machine during the sessions. There is no other formal structuring of the situation or set of injunctions given apart from a

49

statement by the therapist at the beginning of the first session to the effect that 'perhaps we could discuss what led to X's coming into hospital' or, alternatively, 'perhaps we could discuss what seems to have been the trouble here'.

It has been our experience that this sort of family investigation, coupled with observations in the ward-group interactions, can make intelligible those 'symptoms' regarded, in the conventional view of schizophrenia, as being most absurd or meaningless. By this means we can usually discover the method in madness, the secret sense of nonsense.

To illustrate these remarks we shall consider the case of Eric V. The family investigation here consisted of twenty-five interviews with Eric and both his parents, two interviews with his parents on their own, one interview with Eric and father, one with Eric and mother, one with Eric and his younger sister Jean, one with sister alone, two with mother alone, and two with father alone. There are also a number of observations on his interaction with others in the ward community.

Eric V was admitted to our mental hospital, as a legally detained patient, for the first time in 1960, when he was nineteen years of age. The clinical 'mental state' examination at that time included statements to the effect that he was impulsive and unco-operative and that he showed 'thought disorder' and could give no coherent account of himself apart from vehement denials that there was anything wrong with him and demands that he be allowed immediately to return to the University in Wales which he had left of his own accord two days earlier. He would (in his pyjamas) make wild dashes from the ward which were physically restrained by the nurses and by large doses of sedation. He had ideas of references and aural hallucinations: he believed that people, even those who did not know him, looked down on him and called him 'soft'. He believed he heard staff telling him that he had no right to be in hospital and that he should go home – which he tried forcibly to do despite staff restraint.

The immediate background to his admission was that a week earlier, a fortnight before the end of his first term, he had telephoned his father to announce without explanation that he was returning to his home in London from the university. He did in fact commence the train journey home but got off at a station half way and attempted to hitch-hike back to the university. He appeared obviously distressed and confused and was picked up by the police who put him on a train to London.

He arrived at his parents' home very tired and hungry. According to his father he was quite 'rational' but not prepared to talk about himself. His mother welcomed him but he walked straight past her, brusquely brushing her aside. Immediately afterwards, however, he contradicted this gesture of rejection by turning and hugging and kissing her. Later that evening he said he wanted to return to the university and refused to go to bed despite persuasion. His parents, feeling unable to deal with this situation, called in the family doctor, who gave him a sedative. He went to bed but later came downstairs weeping, asking 'What can I do?' His father assured him that he had done the right thing in coming home where he could get help with his problems. Eric, however, denied that he needed help of any sort. He slept well that night but the next morning, although the doctor had advised him to spend the day in bed, he again announced his intention to return to the university. He shocked his family by saying that he hated his mother. It was at this stage that his doctor called in the Mental Welfare Officer, who arranged, with the formal authority of the doctor, for his admission to the mental hospital 'just for a short rest'.

When Eric's father saw the doctor alone shortly after Eric's admission to the ward, he was extremely distraught. He said that he had never really known his son, that Eric had always longed for affection but had always been diffident about accepting it, especially from him. He said that Eric had never wanted to be fondled as a child and had always shunned any form of affection that seemed in any way 'effeminate'. It was a terrible shock to hear him say that day that he hated his mother. His father seemed anxious to hear not that Eric would 'get better' but that he and, somewhat more vaguely, his wife had nothing to reproach themselves about in relation to the boy's 'illness'. Mr V did not know anything about what had gone on at the university and the only 'evidence of illness' that he produced was (*a*) that Eric had been somewhat extravagantly interested in politics over the last year, (*b*) that he had returned home from university for no apparent reason, (*c*) that he said, on arriving home, that he wanted to return to the university but did not want to discuss the matter with his parents, (*d*) that he said he hated his mother. Eric's home life, according to his father, was generally happy and 'better than average'.

In the first family group meeting during Eric's first week in hospital the interaction assumed a fairly rigid form which persisted during the next two meetings: Eric was firmly defined as the 'sick one'. Father adopted an inquisitorial attitude in which he would legalistically interrogate Eric regarding his symptoms, very much as in the conventional psychiatric mental state examination. Eric was sick; the doctors and his parents were going to help him get better; he should co-operate, have confidence in these good people, stay in hospital, and accept treatment (Eric was at this time making repeated efforts to leave the ward and go home or back to the university). During these sessions mother remained very much in the background, occasionally confirming father's pronouncements.

As these early meetings progressed father adopted an increasingly moralistic tone. It was no longer clear to what extent Eric was being regarded as ill and to what extent as bad (lazy, uncooperative). Father would point to various small resemblances between his son and himself and, in various contexts, gave his son repeated injunctions to identify with him, to cope with social situations in the same way that he did – after all he had had the same difficulties. It became increasingly evident that in these sessions father was trying to present to Eric in a highly condensed form the sort of fathering that is accorded most small boys throughout their childhood. Had Eric lacked this experience of a father before? In the third to fifth sessions this became more and more clearly affirmed by mother, who finally mounted a full-scale attack on father in terms of his never having made himself available to the family as a person. When Eric was twelve his father went to India, where he remained for eighteen months. This absence was regarded by mother as an extreme threat to the integrity of the family and she exposed her husband as never having made a serious decision about the family: they went to India to join father and it was mother's decision which led the whole family to return to England and settle down. Eric joined in this attack on his father, accusing him of evading his responsibilities. Father presented only a very feeble defence of himself, but then countered the attack with assertions to the effect that his wife had over-mothered Eric and had never allowed him any independent movement.

At this stage the parents were interviewed without Eric. It was clear that in between sessions a great deal had been going on between them and now they felt that their relationship, and consequently the family, was in great danger. The relationship, mother said, had never been secure owing mainly to father's 'withdrawal' from the family. Father, while accepting blame for this, complained that mother was putting the entire responsibility for Eric's illness on to him. The original façade of a united family with a son who had just 'got ill' for no apparent reason began rapidly to break down. Mother expressed her own fears of a mental breakdown and said that she was in fact ill now 'through always taking other people's troubles on to myself'. Important further information regarding the background of the parents was now forthcoming. Father had had a working-class background in the North of England. There had never been a spark of kindness in his family, he had lived in fear of his father, who drank excessively, and an older brother. He had worked himself up to a skilled engineering job with a good salary. Mother had had a lower middle-class background in the Midlands. Her father was totally withdrawn from the family. Her mother, a teacher, domineered over the children and had no time for housework or the comforts of the family. She did not want any of her children to marry, she wanted companions: 'My mother was more adapted for a public life . . . not at all domesticated, we were

53

just visitors in our home.' Mrs V felt that her mother always resented her having Eric. She herself felt that she 'lacked mothering instinct' when she had him and it was clear that in her relationship with her own mother she had not been able to build up any attitude of self-esteem or confidence in her adult feminine capacities. In the year before Eric's birth her younger sister had had an illegitimate baby and the V's had had to arrange for its adoption ... 'She had to give up her baby when I had mine.' Her mother was very upset by this situation and Eric's presence was painful to Mrs V's sister, who packed up her bags and left. Her mother and family completely ignored Mrs V's baby. Eric had a normal birth and was breast fed for eleven weeks but his mother then gave it up because she felt he was not gaining weight. She 'worked to the book' with him and his physical progress was then good. When his sister was born four years later the situation in the family was much happier. Mrs V's mother had gone off with the younger sister and the V's had their own house and felt much more secure.

Eric did very well academically at school but never really had a friend outside his family. He had always been extremely shy with women and had never been out with a girl. He won a state scholarship and intended to study modern languages at the university. His parents would have liked him to go to Cambridge but he failed the entrance examination. His father had bought him various left-wing periodicals to help him in the general knowledge examination and it was from this reading that Eric's 'preoccupation' with politics and nuclear disarmament commenced. In fact, not only had his interest in politics been determined by his parents but the limits of this interest were also defined for him by them – when he told a local shopkeeper that he should boycott South African goods, his parents let him know that they felt things were going too far. When he failed to obtain a place in Cambridge the next best was the university in Wales – in the same city in which his mother had trained in domestic science. His father was very concerned that Eric should have the opportunities which he himself had missed. This much sounds quite in line with social norms, but many facts apart from those briefly mentioned here supported the view that Eric's future was being precisely and rigidly mapped out for him by his family to fit in with the past experiences and present needs of his parents. Eric was, to an unusual degree, to be the vehicle in which his parents lived out vicariously, to a gratifying conclusion, all their past unfulfilled wishes and frustrated needs. There was very little room left for him to be anything or anyone on his own. He found it virtually impossible to see himself as 'myself' – 'myself' for him always had the existential structure of 'yourself'; in more philosophical language his being-for-the-others (object being) had ontological precedence for him over his being-for-himself (subject being). At the height of his confusion about 'who' he was, when he was leaving the university to return home, he wrote a 'thought-disordered' letter to the university authorities with a usage of pronominal forms which well illustrates this subject-object confusion:

'Eric has decided to leave and wishes to say how very sorry he is for the way he has treated everyone here at the university. I am lost. I must act. I am going. So, please once again, Professors, Lecturers, post-graduates, under-graduates, sorry. I most truly am, Yours faithfully, Spoilt Kid, Eric V.'

In another very apologetic letter to his tutor he signed himself 'self-centred, Eric V'.

A central feature in Eric's history was his 'arriving' and 'departing', his 'inexplicable' decision to return home from the university followed immediately by his wish to go back there. Also, while in hospital, he made repeated attempts to leave in order sometimes, he said, to go home, sometimes to return to the university (on two occasions he went home from hospital without leave but on both occasions he promptly wished to return to the hospital). In one of the early sessions the following exchange took place:

DR B: . . . Well, yesterday, for instance, the main theme seemed to be that you wanted to leave the hospital.

ERIC: Yes, well, I do feel that really. My staying here wouldn't be of any use to myself. Or anybody else really. I feel I've got to take some positive action really . . . positive action of . . . of my own, which nobody else has arranged for me. I feel I've got to go back to the university.

DR B: Mm.

ERIC: I must go back to university straight away and get stuck into my work there.

FATHER: Do you feel, Eric, that you are . . . you'd be able to get stuck into your work . . . at the present time.

ERIC: (4 seconds) Well, my mind doesn't feel very strong somehow.

FATHER: Well, there has been a distinct improvement since you came here. Don't you think, acting on Dr B's advice, Dr C's advice, that it might be better to reconcile yourself to remaining for a time longer until you do feel more capable of tackling your studies when you go back to university.

MOTHER: What do you think about that, doctor?

DR B: Well . . . I . . . Eric and I have discussed this quite a lot, and time and again of course Eric has repeated that he feels that he must take some positive step himself. This is what you said, isn't it?

ERIC: Yes.

DR B: That you must get back to university. I feel that . . . that probably this difference in point of view is what we ought to try and examine. Your parents feel that you should stay here, and you feel you must go to university, and work. . . .

ERIC: Well, I think . . . I think it's what I feel I ought to do is important really. I've got . . . I've got to take . . . I mean I mustn't lean on other people. I feel I must . . . I must act independently, not have things done for me.

MOTHER: That's quite true, Eric. But we want you to feel that – er when you go back to university there are two things that are going to be essential to feel – that you're making progress when you get back, and that you're pursuing your studies successfully, and another thing, that you feel quite happy about, let us say, the people you meet there. You mustn't have these ideas that they're disparaging you in any way. You must feel confident of their approval and – otherwise if you don't feel like that, you're going to have another setback, aren't you? And do you think that those two conditions would be fulfilled if you went back to university. Do you feel confident that people will ... are wanting you and building on you, and you wouldn't have any of these unpleasant feelings about being wanted there. How do you feel about it? (4 seconds) ... I assure you, you are wanted there, without any doubt whatever.

ERIC: I don't feel that people – wouldn't think about ... think like that about me.

MOTHER: Do you feel confident about ... that, that's as it should be.

ERIC: In the light of my behaviour they might possibly not think very highly of me. My – er – departure from university and so on can't have shown me up in a very good – shown me up very well at all.

MOTHER: I assure you, Eric, that when you go back there it will be just like turning over on to a clean page. And you'll make a completely fresh start there ...

FATHER: Yes, you'll have to credit them with understanding, that you left ... the circumstances under which you left were that you were disturbed to the point where you couldn't do anything else. And they'll look upon it, as it is, as a sickness. When you get back they'll ...

ERIC: I was definitely unwell when I came here, was I?

FATHER: Yes, I think you were.

ERIC: Mm. I wonder if I was.

FATHER: And Eric, coming to this question, this desire that you have ... you do mention, to be independent, and to act independently. It's a very commendable and admirable – er – desire – there's no doubt about it. And – er – you – we all did long to achieve our independence. But the more we – when we do acquire this independence we do at the same time realize how dependent we are also on others. You can't be absolutely and completely independent of other people anyhow. You've got to have some dependence on others. I mean, even to the extent – you take the simplest things – you get on a bus, you're dependent on the driver that he's taking you on the right course. . . . Modern life with gregarious existence is quite impossible without dependence on others.

ERIC: You're not dependent on them to get away.

FATHER: Where that dependence begins and ends is another point.

ERIC: You're dependent on him for taking you where you want to go, not for taking you off the bus.

FATHER: Well, it's only a simple illustration – a very simple illustration.

ERIC: Dependent on him taking you there, yet.

MOTHER: Well, you're quite capable of deciding things for yourself, Eric, and it seems to me that the true crux of the matter is will you feel quite happy about the company you're in, that you won't have any idea that people are not wanting you there. . . . If you feel happy about that it would make such a difference.

Eric states the need for him to carry out some significant autonomous act. His parents interpose the opaque datum of his illness, in particular his ideas of reference, and we shall return to this point they make. The truth is, however, that Eric had never carried out a single independent act in his life. Everything he had done had had to fit in with and be directed by a complex system of external and internalized, spoken and unspoken parental injunctions. Eric had never gone to the university at all: his parents had sent him there. True, he had passively absorbed and reproduced for examinations a certain mass of knowledge, and he had done this very well, but always in the context of his parents' projects for him, never in pursuit of a project of his own. The mystery of his return from the university becomes wholly intelligible if we see it not as a strange unreasoning act, but as a negativity, a non-act or the reverse side of a positive act, by which he set the stage for his first big autonomous action. He came home from the university to which he had been sent *in order to go to the university*. As soon as he arrived home he wanted to return – but return by his own choice. *He* was going to the university for the first time. To do this he had to disinvolve himself from the engulfing parental concern that awaited him, he brushed his mother aside and would not speak to his parents or let them 'help' him. It was this autonomous assertion of himself that led to his coming into hospital. His dramatic assumption of free personal agency threatened the whole structure of the family's existence: it had to be invalidated by the invention of an illness. If he was ill the whole thing became a neutral process which had happened to him. The disturbing praxis, the intention, and the act evaporated.

Eric did not take this lying down, however. He persistently tried to leave hospital and never fully accepted the invalidating attribution of illness made by his family and inevitably confirmed by the quasi-medical dependency situation in the hospital (throughout his first admission he was in the general admission ward of the hospital; it was only during his second admission that he came into the unit). The whole situation became more complex, however, in so far as his parents persistently invited him to assert himself independently in all sorts of ways while remaining impervious to his own attempt to do so. If he were to take up his parents' invitation he would fall into a trap because he would then once again be merely following their direction. The liberation he was offered was in fact a Trojan horse. To act freely entailed his submission to the injunction to be free: freedom and unfreedom were finally equated.

The attributions of illness, apart from the 'irrational' coming and going, rest mainly on Eric's inexplicable ideas that people were making remarks to the effect that he was a useless, self-centred, lazy, sexually abnormal person. Some of the following exchanges may render these ideas less inexplicable:

(Eric is talking about his lack of confidence and inability to concentrate.)

MOTHER: And have you tried to account for it all?

ERIC: No . . . I put it down to selfishness, you see. Self-centredness.

MOTHER: You haven't tried to think whether it could have been anything else?

ERIC: Well just recently I think it might have been the result of my masturbation.

MOTHER: Mm. . . .

ERIC: You se. . . .

MOTHER: Mm. . . .

FATHER: You mentioned this to me for the first time the other week, Eric, and it obviously seemed to be worrying you, this matter of masturbation. Er . . . I think . . . and I know from my own experience, as I've already told you, I think pretty well every, every . . . er . . . man anyway, tries it out at some time or other. And again I . . . I . . . I've read and I'm quite prepared to believe that, er, that er, if it becomes . . . if . . . if . . . if . . . you lose your self-respect to the extent of practising it regularly, then it can have a very deleterious effect on your general health. I mean, it's something . . . it's something really . . . it is something that's . . . it's more disrespectful, it's yourself really, I think. And for that reason it, it can undermine your . . . your confidence.

MOTHER: Don't you think a lot of these excesses are a reflection of . . . of . . . these tensions . . . and perhaps a period that you might be going through where you're exposed to other strains, and the . . . these excesses are symptoms, and . . . I remember you talking about buying a lot of sweets. And there's only one time in my life when I was exposed to a phenomenal strain, in fact it was the very first job I ever had in my life and I spent all my money at the sweet shop, something I'd never done before or since. And that was a symptom you see. It was a kind of compensation for the strain I was undergoing. And I think masturbation is another of these excesses that is a symptom of stresses and strains. It's never the cause.

ERIC: When I was at the university, I didn't masturbate at all in anybody's bed . . . well . . . I did once or twice . . . yes . . . once or twice at the beginning. Then I did get over it, really got over it. But then I went buying chocolates and Mars bars . . .

FATHER: I think this masturbation is a phase, you know, that most people pass through at some time or other, Eric. I believe it is, I don't know, I mean there may be . . . I may be quite wrong but I've got an idea that it is a phase that . . . people pass through. But there again, Eric, you got to . . .

ERIC: I've been shy of girls all the time, haven't I? I mean, I've had an unhealthy relationship with girls . . . I've never mixed with girls because I've been shy.

MOTHER: Do you admire them from a distance, Eric?

ERIC: I admire them as individuals. . . . I just admire what they do and so on.

FATHER: But from a sexual point of view do you regard them as . . . I mean, do you regard them as being something, you know, very sweet and demure and desirable and romantic?

ERIC: Not now.

FATHER: Not now. But you have done?

ERIC: I have done on occasions.

FATHER: Yes, I think it's a pretty healthy aspect of the female, you know, a pretty healthy view of the female. I know I did, and I think most young fellows do [3 seconds]. But you know again, coming back to that question (that's all right Eric) . . . [Eric cries]. . . . Can you say what's upsetting you particularly. . . .

ERIC: No . . . [tearfully] I have periods at times, on occasions when I'm sitting in the rest room down in the . . . you know . . . the ward there, when I'm listening to music. There are certain chords, you know, tunes that suddenly make me cry.

FATHER: I've experienced that countless times, Eric, a

particularly moving passage of music brings the tears to my eyes, and I don't think that's uncommon at all.

MOTHER: We were looking at a film, weren't we, on television the other night, and I couldn't help it, it was so beautiful. And I cried. It's very very natural, Eric. We all need, I think, these outlets.

FATHER: Do you feel at the present time, Eric, it's . . . there's anything of self-pity in your crying? Feeling sorry for yourself?

ERIC: . . . I feel it's just pent-up emotion.

FATHER: Well, we've all suffered from them, and I've wept these last two weeks I'll tell you, when I came to see Dr B when you came in. I couldn't help but weep, and it was my, you know, an emotional upset that I just couldn't restrain the tears.

MOTHER: It's one of nature's ways.

In this passage it is simultaneously asserted by the parents that masturbation is normal and that it is a symptom and something that *could* be the cause of Eric's lack of confidence. Father seems quite impervious to Eric's grief over his lack of any masculine identification and rapidly goes on to make the implicit attribution (framed as a question) of self-pity. This is one of the things that Eric 'irrationally' thinks 'other people' think about him. As with all these derogatory attributions guilt usually inhibits Eric from identifying his parents as the 'other people'.

A frequent move on the parents' part is to disarm criticism by inviting it:

FATHER: Well, you know . . . I've often been very exasperated at Eric's – er – disinterestedness and what I've thought to be . . . an inability to – er . . . ? . . . that I expected, you know. And I . . . I've made disparaging remarks about his ability to grasp anything, and to show a bit of common sense, things like that, you know. And told him he was dumb and goodness knows what. You know – and he's obviously, you know, felt some reaction, but he's never expressed anything, he's never come back at me. I remember saying to him at one time – My God, Eric, I only wish you'd lose your temper with me sometimes when I . . . er . . . talk like this to you. I wish you'd get it out of you and attack me – you know – in retaliation. But he . . . he . . . didn't. He used to . . . never has done. I don't know whether it's an exaggerated respect for me . . . or what it is. But I've often felt that I've been very very unworthy in my – you know – in some of the things I've said to him.

DR C: What do you think about this, Eric, what your father's just said?

ERIC: Yes, he has said things on occasions which have hurt me very much. But . . . it's difficult to . . . to put this . . . this may have had a cause . . . you know, started from . . . this may have been started by something which – er – which may have thrown me into this condition. And now I can't remember where and when it started.

FATHER: Well, I've felt ashamed at some of the things I've said to you, you know, and yet I've thought, well most people, all of us have these things said to us, and what we have to learn to do, and it's a pretty painful process, as we grow up, is to put them in the right place and on balance to weigh things up, weigh up whether those things were said in the heat of the moment, whether they were really sincere, whether they, you know, when they're measured against the, the complimentary things that are said and the expressions of respect and devotion, *love* even, etc., whether they deserve a place, you know, in your mind. All the hard things that have been said to me, you know I told you the other day, when we had this discussion before . . .

The effect of father's stratagems is that Eric, while acknowledging that he has been hurt by father's remarks, is completely alienated from his feelings of anger in response to them. He ponders, mystified, about some sort of unrelated 'condition' or process in himself.

As the group progresses, the relation between Eric's 'hallucinated' remarks and his father's actual attributions becomes clearer. Father accepts more and more responsibility for this and moves to a more exposed position in the family where mother confronts him with a view of himself totally opposed to his previous self-conception:

ERIC: That's how I was feeling at the university, though. I felt that everybody had a down on me.

MOTHER: But you didn't have that feeling before you went?

ERIC: I felt that everybody had a down on me then.

FATHER: You told me, Eric, that . . .

ERIC: . . . sort of staring at me, you know.

FATHER: Mm.

ERIC: . . . and hearing people saying things about me, stupid . . . you know . . . he's insulted everybody in the university . . . these things I remember quite distinctly.

MOTHER: Do you believe them now, that they were really heard?

ERIC: Oh yes, I believe they were really said. I remember them quite distinctly. And . . . that they really hurt.

FATHER: You cared about it?

MOTHER: Of course he did.

FATHER: Yes.

ERIC: Then I tried to apologise to one or two people . . . you know . . . I thought I'd insulted, and I tried to patch up things as best I could.

MOTHER: Do you remember what you said when your results came through in the State scholarship? [3 seconds]

ERIC: Yes.

MOTHER: Do you know something you said? It proved something [2 seconds]. You don't remember now?

FATHER: Go on, tell him.

ERIC: 'That proves I can do it,' or something. . . . What did I say?

MOTHER: You said, 'It's proved to Dad that I'm not stupid'.

You said, 'I wanted to get the State scholarship to prove to Dad that I wasn't stupid.'

FATHER: I rather think, Eric, you know, that my accusations of stupidity at times have . . . have really upset you, and er . . . I don't know how I can make amends. I mean . . . it's not . . . I don't feel that . . . you know . . . I've accused . . . And you seem to have some doubts as to whether what I've said has been sincere at times. You know, when I've tried to put a point across to you and said, honestly Eric, I really and truly believe that from the depths of my heart, you know and I've felt, you know that I haven't got it across to you. I wonder if that's associated in any way with the . . . the er . . . frivolity that I've been guilty of . . . or guilty of, I don't think I should say *guilty* of it – indulged in at home, from time to time. When I've thought it should make somebody laugh and instead of that it's made somebody cry.

MOTHER: But we were having a talk the other day, weren't we, about . . . er . . . how can you convince anybody of their regard for you. Just saying it isn't enough. That is not convincing. Do you remember us having this talk? And I said you can only convince anybody of your regard for them by proving to them that you think about them, and that you're anxious to preserve at least some of their interests, and that when you're not in their company you think about them, and you remember some of the things in which they take part, and you admitted that you are a bit sort of lax in this respect. I mean for instance, with Jean, she's been going to a club on Wednesday nights, hasn't she, for some time. And one evening she'd got her coat on ready to go and you said, 'Oh hello, going out?' And she said, 'Yes, it's the club.' 'Oh, oh yes.' You know. Well, I mean, if you'd become more familiar, if you'd familiarized yourself a bit more with her doings, you would have realized where she was going. But I mean that is rather typical of you, isn't it? I mean, I've been going to things that have been even talked about, you know, something sort of special, and you've come home and made no mention of it. And I'll say, 'Oh, I went so and so.' 'Oh yes, I remember now, you said you were going.' You're a bit remote from people's lives. And when you're remote from people's lives like that it rather tends to give the impression that you're not really interested in them. And whether that is the kind of impression, you know, you've conveyed to Eric as well, er . . . I suppose we've all shared in this experience, haven't we? Jean, me, Eric, we've all shared in this experience. And I have made strenuous efforts haven't I, at times, to draw you back into the family group and get you to take a little more interest in us. To be one of four, instead of three and one. And you've said to me, 'Oh well it's easier for you, the children come home first and they tell it all to you first, and I only hear things second hand.'

FATHER: Well, that's a fact really.

MOTHER: But at the same time opportunities abound to interest yourself in the affairs of the family, if you're sufficiently interested to take advantage of them, and you are a bit like that.

FATHER: Yes, I am perhaps a bit of an isolationist myself . . . mentally.

MOTHER: And then if you are isolationist it's terribly difficult to convince people that you really are – you care about them, you're proud of them, and then when the onslaught comes, you say something that you really didn't mean, they've no defences against it. They've built up no defences against it you see – and you're extremely vulnerable to these attacks when you haven't had those periods of confidence in somebody to help you to sustain that.

DR C: What do you think, Eric, about your father's 'isolationism'?

ERIC: I think it may be something I've inherited – I think I have inherited it.

FATHER: You think it is a fact that I am rather like that, rather remote?

ERIC: Er . . . yes. Oh yes, you are.

FATHER: Do you think it was always so?

MOTHER: Not in the family circle anyway.

FATHER: Well, I don't know what the impression is we give to Dr B and Dr C here, but the fact is at home Mum's the talker and I'm the listener, usually. That could generally be said. . . . Mum likes to thrash everything out, get everything discussed and brought to the surface and mauled over and all the rest of it, and I rather tend to think that if a thing's said, when once a thing's said people ought to give you credit for being sincere in what you say and, when once it's said, it's said, and there is no need to repeat it. . . . But of course you say things . . .

MOTHER: . . . New problems are coming up all the time, aren't they? Specially with a growing family. New problems are presenting themselves for . . . by your family, in which you've got to kind of . . . it presents opportunities for . . . not necessarily opportunities . . . but necessity for discussion. Once, I mean, the things you've said, you're not going to think of repeating the same old things over and over again, are you? I mean, Jean at 15, the kind of talk that goes on between you, between her and her parents at 15, is vastly different from what it was at 12 or 10, and so on. Life's changing all the time and new subjects are coming up for discussion.

FATHER: You have found it difficult, Eric, to talk to me at all . . . found it difficult to mention any problem to me, or to talk to me on any old subject for that matter.

ERIC: Yes.

FATHER: Have you felt that whenever we did talk it would be in an argumentative kind of . . . way?

ERIC: Yes.

MOTHER: You're on the defensive from the word go, aren't you. And your way of thinking about things is that attack is the best line of defence. And that's what you do. You go all out to attack, you see, and whittle away your opponent's arguments, and sort of wear him down, you know, with your point of view. And you pride yourself you know, that you've never lost an argument yet.

FATHER: [laughs] That's going far.

ERIC: There may be . . . honestly, Dad, maybe you just can't help it, but he has said terribly heartless things on occasion.

MOTHER: Oh, he has. Terrible.

DR C: He seems to be having the worst of this argument.

FATHER: He does, doesn't he. You know, the virtuous impression I have of myself is that generally speaking I'm quiet, I won't argue, because – or I won't even sometimes express an opinion – because I shall – it will lead to an argument. And the argument will lead to bad feeling. And I have rather regarded myself more or less as a peace-at-any-price kind of individual . . .

MOTHER: Now, now . . .

FATHER: There have been occasions, of course, when we've had arguments, and . . . I can never win an argument at home.

MOTHER: Oh, yes you do.

At the end of this session there is a tense moment. Mother has been speaking of an incident in which she was able to see her mother as a greedy person:

MOTHER: Well, I mean, even if you're angry with people like that, and I think, you know, there does come a time when you can view your parents with that detachment. You know they were good to you in many ways when you were young, and helped you, and I'll admit she helped me and provided a relaxing home, but there comes a time when you view them as adults, and you criticize them as adults, apart from you. You don't see them with rose-coloured spectacles of childhood. And you will come to see us in that way, Eric, the good and the bad in us, without the rose-coloured spectacles of childhood.

ERIC: Well I am . . .

MOTHER: Well, you're entitled to say it.

FATHER: A perfect right to say it.

DR C: What makes you feel that you can't say this then, Eric? Your parents are both inviting you to see them objectively, to say what you feel about them.

ERIC: Well . . . I . . . sentimental affection for them. Restraint from saying what I really feel . . . a sentimental affection for Dad – [long pause] – but I've often really felt I hated him.

FATHER: That's all right, Eric, it's human emotion which we all have, this feeling of hate, and I've argued this point with Mum about this – Mum believes that if you love a person, it's a constant emotion that's always present. And I've argued that that, that . . . at times under the stress of emotion and strain you can actually hate the person you love for a time.

ERIC: No, you can hate a person you love.

FATHER: Not at the same time, not at the same moment . . .

This invitation to criticize his parents is 'double-binding' in the sense that together with the explicit invitation there is an implicit injunction against criticizing what is communicated non-verbally by obvious signals of anxiety from the parents to Eric. Part of the bind has been taken off, however, as father in the preceding exchange has more or less agreed, under pressure from mother, to accept the role of the guilty one. Mother has controlled the situation so that Eric can acknowledge his angry feelings – but only towards his father. Things have developed but the major difficulty remains – Eric's almost total symbiotic dependence on his mother. It will take him another breakdown to begin to learn how to liberate himself from this.

Eric's first stay in hospital was for a period of four and a half months. He was then discharged home and worked in a local light industrial firm for some months. Then he returned to the university, where he completed a fairly successful term.

A few days prior to his return home on vacation, however, he wrote a letter to his father accusing him of laziness and of not having done his duty in the family. He wrote that he hated his father because of his 'laziness' but went on to say that he was writing this letter because really he loved him. His statements in this letter (which was judged to be contradictory and 'confused' by a psychiatrist) were similarly phrased to his mother's earlier accusations against her husband in the family group meetings. Immediately after sending this letter, Eric packed his bags and announced that he was going to South Africa to help the black people in their struggle against the régime (he had no passport and very little money). He was restrained by his fellow-students and admitted on a detention order to a local mental observation ward. He was reported to have said that he heard voices, which he could not identify, telling him to stop thinking of himself, to have concern for others, and to go to South Africa. He was said to have expressed the belief that everyone in the world knew of his every action and was talking about him. He showed 'thought blocking' and was confused and impulsive – attacking the staff and other patients. An acute schizophrenic episode was diagnosed and he was treated with large doses of tranquillizers. When he became a little quieter he was transferred to this hospital – his parents being the prime movers in the transfer.

Once again, in this second breakdown, Eric attempted to assert himself by an autonomous act – his proposed departure to South Africa. But once again, because he had been made to feel that autonomous action was not really his right, and because he had lacked transitional experience from the insecurity-ridden world of his family to experience of the common social reality, he sabotaged himself by proceeding in a manner that was unrealistic by ordinary standards, so drawing on to his head further invalidating attributions of madness. Having produced this situation and having secured his admission to a psychiatric ward, he acted out without restraint his needs to be mothered by 'parent-figures' who would tolerate and, at a certain point, control his aggressive acts – without making him feel guilty about these.

The unidentified 'voices' he was said to have 'heard' accusing him of selfishness were a series of internalizations of statements that had actually been pronounced by his father and recorded by us in the family interactions. Vaguer feelings concerning what 'other people' felt about him, e.g. that he was sexually abnormal and disgusting, had been aroused by feelings which his parents had about him and which were clearly implied by them, if not explicitly stated, in earlier and subsequent family meetings. Eric recognized these internalized statements and feelings as not being his own but to pin them on their true authors was very difficult for him. His father had already been put forward by his mother as a sacrificial offering, and for Eric to identify his father as the source of the denigration was felt by Eric to be tantamount to parricide. So, in the letter to his father he half retracted his accusations. But in the first family group after his return to this hospital he spoke of his father in the past tense – 'you could have been great like Lenin but you were a fascist like Verwoerd' (Eric's lack of transitional social experience made it difficult for him to discover any intermediate human reality between his family and universally known historical personages).

At this stage, however, the family was ready to bring about further changes in itself. The position had altered considerably from the first session in which Eric was so clearly defined as the sick member and his parents by implication as well. First his father and then his mother moved into 'ill' positions. Later Eric moved into a 'strong' position relative to his mother; when she was obviously disturbed he was able to 'treat' her more effectively than father, but at the same time he developed increasing independence of his family. He no longer went home regularly for weekends and succeeded in holding down a job the menial nature of which was totally opposed to his parents' ideas of a suitable career. He made realistic attempts to find a better job, but for some time his therapist in the unit made the mistake of making Eric feel that he should get a better job to please him (the therapist). Once again Eric's future was being determined for him by someone else and it was only after mutual recognition of this fact in the group that Eric could make his own choice reasonably to improve his position. His progress was facilitated by his mother also taking a job which gave her a centre of emotional investment outside the family.

To sum up, we can say that we have tried to follow by a

dialectical method a dialectical movement in the V family group. From the constituted dialectic of Eric's presentation of himself we have moved 'regressively' to the constitutive dialectic (the family praxis), including the observed pattern of family interaction in the present and the past history of the family, tracing an historical pattern through the interrelation of the different accounts of this by the various family members. Then, moving 'progressively', we have outlined a total totalization – the truth of the family and the truth of Eric's breakdown. This truth lies in the desperate tension between, on the one hand, the ultimately untenable position in which his very existence, in his own eyes, became identical with his existence *for others* (his parents), and, on the other, the position in which he attempted to assert his autonomous existence by developing *his own* view of himself and by carrying out *his own* acts. This view and these acts were invalidated for reasons which we have tried to make intelligible.

Certainly the exchanges in family groups call out for psycho-analytic interpretation[1] and to achieve a full comprehension of this segment of the evolution of the V family, we would have to understand the interrelating of the phantasy-systems of its members. We have, however, excluded this mode of studying the interactions in order that we might bring clearly into view the complex interrelation of acts and intentions – the interrelation of decision-systems. Without this latter framework of understanding, 'pure' psycho-analytic work may flounder far from the central issue – Eric's progressive choice of himself in the face of the choices the others make about him.

---

[1] There are certain obvious psycho-analytic give-aways such as Eric's reference to 'Mars bars' on p. 61. The implications of interpretation in this situation of total involvement, however, are infinitely complex and should not be made in terms suggested by two-person psycho-analytic experience.

CHAPTER IV

The Invalid, his Family, and the Ward

In the light of the ideas presented in the preceding chapters, I felt a clear need to produce a psychiatric or, rather, anti-psychiatric situation in which people would not be invalidated or violated beyond the point which they had already attained in these respects at the moment of entering the hospital.

Before one could think of producing a relatively non-invalidatory situation of this nature, however, one had to review whatever tentative signs of progress in this direction already existed. In particular it was necessary to examine fairly exhaustively, in theory and in practice, the 'therapeutic community'. This term has ornamented various projects that range from the relatively 'far out' to perfectly ordinary wards in perfectly ordinary mental hospitals. What, we must inquire, are the origins, of the therapeutic community, its present limits, and its future possibilities?

Perhaps one of the earliest therapeutic communities was the community of the *Therapeutae* that existed in pre-Christian times in Egypt. The origins of this community, described by Philo in *De vita contemplativa* (A.D. 25), are lost in prehistory but we do know a little about the communities themselves. We should note the relation of the two meanings of the Greek word *therapeuein*, to heal, and to serve, since by a curious reversal of roles in our epoch those who are to be healed are not in fact those who have to be served in any but an implicitly derogatory sense. Instead they have to serve or at least to serve time. In the community of

73

the Therapeutae the members of the community lived in some-times quite remotely scattered houses – near enough to afford protection from invaders but not so close as to disturb essential solitude. Each house contained a meditation room and the community member would spend the whole week in solitary meditation. On one fixed day, however, the whole community would pray, sing, and eat in each other's presence.

To walk into some places styled therapeutic communities in the present-day psychiatric world is to experience a despairing realization that one is in the midst of people who for the most part are lost in their own outer worlds and the outer worlds of others. They live a sterile 'emptied-out' form of group existence. There is a constant struggle to invent, and then re-invent, a sort of interpersonal technology for handling one another in this externalized manner and the protagonists seem to be deprived of even the slight taste of futility that some awareness of this collective project would bring. One longs for someone actually to *do* something, to express something real of himself, something from his existential inside.

The central idea by which one must assess the worthwhileness of a form of social organization proclaiming itself to be a thera-peutic community is one that defines a certain relation between self and others. This relation, I have concluded, must be such that in the total structure *solitude* as enriching inwardness is maintained inviolate, while at the same time there is community in the sense of a contact between the inner worlds as well as the outer worlds of persons. By inner worlds I mean the freedom or intentional core of a person, the source of all his acts finally issuing as objectifiable behaviour, that is the outer world of the person. In other words, the aim of a community that would be truly healing, a community of freedoms, must be to produce a situation in which people can be with each other in such a way that they can actually leave each other alone.

In our age we are totally conditioned to interference from others, we gravely lack the conditions for the full development of the capacity to be alone. For most of us the rot of interference commences in the cradle and does not end before the grave. It requires considerable artifice to escape this process even momentarily. And yet I believe that it is only on the basis of an adequate capacity to be alone that we can find a true way of being with others. We have to rediscover the lost meaning of the Taoist principle of *wu wei*, the principle of non-action, but a positive non-action that requires an effort of self-containment, an effort to cease interference, to 'lay off' other people and give them and oneself a chance.

The psychiatric therapeutic community, however, does not, in general, spring from this sort of protest against interference. In some statements of principle there is an emphasis rather on time-economy and an implicitly quantified communication matrix, e.g. the therapeutic community as a solution to the problem of 'the other twenty-three hours' (the rest of the day when the patient's session with the doctor is over), 'feedback' from peripheral transactions to central groups in order to limit wastage of significant communications, and so on. The pioneering work of Maxwell Jones (1952), which established a prototype for the therapeutic community, is well known, as is that of Wilmer (1958) and Artiss (1962), for instance, who have run 'acute' reception units more or less on these lines in the U.S. Navy and Army respectively.

The task I chose, however, was to develop a unit specifically orientated to the problem of young people who had recently acquired the label 'schizophrenia', in which the approach would be based on an understanding of schizophrenia not as a disease-entity, but as a certain more or less specifiable set of personal-interactional patterns; schizophrenia, that is to say, not as something happening *in* a person but rather something between persons. We should attempt, in fact, to do without what Don Jackson has described as 'that curse of modern psychiatry, the identified patient'.

The therapeutic groups, I had decided on the basis of previous experience, would not be analytical groups in which the words and actions of patients are interpreted reductively with a view to the long-term working-through of conflicts. This was not only because patients would stay in the unit for, usually, not more than a few months, but also because I regarded such an approach as inappropriate to the type of problem called 'hospitalized acute schizophrenia'. Essentially this latter situation is one of intense mystification about virtually everything that goes on between the identified patient and the other persons involved in the episode. Demystification of these issues is necessary before one can think in terms of recommending either two-person or group-analytic psychotherapy or psycho-analysis.

Of course transference 'happens' in the groups in the unit, not only in the sense that the therapist is treated as a parent-figure, but also, in the sense of whole-family transference where types of relating and patterns of interacting peculiar to the family are repeated by the patient in the therapeutic group, invoking the collusion of others in the group. Two people, for instance, join together as a parental team electing a third person as their child. They then practise techniques of confusing the 'child', undermining his perceptions of himself and of them, perhaps to the extent of producing a 'psychotic reaction' in him unless the therapist intervenes. In fact they are reproducing, as a means of clarifying their own positions, patterns of interaction which they know only too well in their own families where they are on the receiving end. The only way of handling this sort of situation is by an intervention that makes the whole process explicit. Such an intervention is in fact a metacommunication, a communication about the sort of communication going on in the triadic sub-group which no one in the sub-group is himself able to make and thereby escape the destructive situation.

Transference and projection, then, are always present, but we must be cautious regarding interpretation. What happens when we try to interpret reductively an irreducible fact? We must bear in mind the possibility that when a patient says his mother is driving him mad, he may be correct, at least in the sense that his mother's attributions of madness in him may dominate the whole pseudo-medical set-up of his being a patient in hospital. Certain

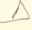

psycho-analytic writers working in a monadic situation, seeing the patient in isolation from his human environment, seem sometimes fatally to limit themselves in this respect. Rosenfeld (1955, p. 191) for instance writes:

'In some papers on schizophrenia particularly by American writers like Pious and Fromm-Reichmann the mother's hostile and 'schizophrenogenic' attitude has been stressed. The mother in this case seems to have been unconsciously hostile to the patient and the patient's illness increased her guilty feelings. But we ought not to forget that in all mental disturbances there is a close inter-relationship between external factors acting as trauma and internal ones which are determined mostly by heredity. In our analytic approach we know that it is futile and even harmful to the progress of an analysis to accept uncritically the patient's attempts to blame the external environment for his illness. We generally find that there exists a great deal of distortion of external factors through projection and we have to help the patient to understand his phantasies and reactions to external situations until he becomes able to differentiate between his phantasies and external reality.'

This 'close inter-relationship' runs the risk of being in fact a confusion. Admitting the obvious probability that the patient distorts external factors through projection, how do we then go on to help the patient to differentiate between his phantasies and 'external reality' if we have not the remotest idea what the external reality is? The answer might be to have a look and see; and this is where observations in the family group are not only helpful but essential. Family group meetings consisting of the therapist, the patient, and his nuclear family, or at least one or both parents, should therefore be a regular part of any therapeutic programme.

The aim must be to comprehend the present behaviour of the patient, his 'schizophrenic' presentation of himself, in terms of both a 'vertical' and a 'horizontal' complexity. The vertical complexity concerns his development in the family, going back to the familial origins of *his* parents. The horizontal complexity concerns his interactions here and now with the patients and staff in the unit and with his parents when they visit and when he goes home on weekends. By this means we would be able to ascertain precisely the forms of invalidation the person has encountered and by what failures in his own strategy of living he has become prey to them. We would also become aware of the peculiar tension of his need for some sort of renewal of himself. If we could both sense this need and then provide the right human context for its fulfilment, the patient might find a personal justification for being in the ward community rather than simply react to the needs of massified society temporarily to dispose of him.

Despite the immense practical difficulties encountered when trying to put this into practice, the situation that I felt to be necessary can be quite simply stated. One needs to be allowed to go to pieces and one needs to be helped to come together again. I say 'one' very deliberately, since, although for some people going to pieces is enforced by those who surround them, the need is present in every one of us. We need to be perpetually renewed, born again from the ashes of a temporary state of disintegration or death. I am not speaking here, of course, of biological birth and death, nor am I speaking metaphorically. What I am referring to is existential coming into the world, the world of other persons and of things, and of departing from this world in a very particular sense. By departure I mean a separation from my being in the sense of my being-here, placed in the midst of other beings and seeming to share the 'quality' of being with them. The separation is necessitated by a certain realization in me, one implication of which is that being can never be, or even appear to be, a quality or attribute in this sense. In this realization I apprehend not the being but the nothing that I am, since my departure is not without direction and *my* non-being is what I have departed towards. My non-being is a particular, circumscribed nothingness. Being, *my* being, is at the rim of this nothingness. But this particular nothingness diffuses into the general nothingness or void, or a-voided being.

There is a bipolar diffusion of myself into the general plenitude of being and into pure, a-particular nothing. My concrete and specific existence resides at the infinitesimal point of transition from one pole to the other. This is the non-metaphorical or relatively non-metaphorical ontological model, but there are certain metaphorical models that may assist communication.

One such metaphorical model is that of Ygdrasil the world-tree in North European mythology. Ygdrasil is most familiar to us but the idea of the world-tree is an almost universal image among people trying to grasp their spiritual reality. It is quite central to shamanism, which although geographically located in recent times mainly in Siberia, Mongolia, Manchuria, once extended to many parts of the world with evidence of a temporal extension into prehistoric times. In certain shamanistic tribes corpses were exposed to the elements on biers at the tops of trees, but more importantly one must note the ascension ritual itself which is the real essence of shamanism.

The shaman was the spiritual leader of these tribes. The elements of his identity included those of priest, psychotherapist, witch-doctor, magician, madman. His special powers were sometimes regarded as the result of hereditary transmission but usually there was a process of initiation through which the future shaman was guided by a special type of denizen of the spirit world who became embodied for this purpose. During these preparatory rites the shaman learned to have vivid experiences of his own future corpse and to experience in an extreme of agony his own dismemberment and bodily dissolution.

It is noteworthy that dreams in which one experiences one's own dismemberment in many cases precede either a psychotic breakdown or a creative period of spiritual development – a period of either breakdown or breakthrough. The distinction between these two alternatives resides mainly in the supervening processes of social invalidation, but these may be decisively destructive. Psychotic experience may, with correct guidance, lead to a more advanced human state but only too often is converted by psychiatric interference into a state of arrest and stultification of the person.

When the shaman was fully equipped for his spiritual role, the tribe would gather around him to benefit vicariously from his repeated experiences of, first, possession by the spirits of dead ancestors and other ultra-mundane beings, then a separation of an astral self from his body. The astral self would ascend to the higher world and then return to re-animate its body. This fact of ec-stasis entailed an experience of ecstasy in the shaman which was aided by his beating an oval drum and his wearing deer-antlers and emblems of other animals, in particular birds. Through their vicarious, 'projective' participation in this experience, the other members of the tribe would benefit from a *therapeusis*. They would have some reflected experience of the shaman's possession, existential death, dissolution, ec-stasis and ascent, descent and en-stasis. Therapeusis here meant renewal of each person through death and rebirth achieved by these miraculous means within one life-span.

In the community of officially 'psychotic' people I shall describe in this book, this form of renewal was enacted repeatedly although usually on a scale less formally extended than in the Shamanistic rite.

The needs of people vary widely. Some people are brought up in families that function anti-dialectically in the sense that they can *only* bring up their children – they cannot achieve the position in which their children are both brought up *and* bring themselves up, with the implied decisive act of separation. In such families one finds that one or more of the children are progressively pushed into a final, extreme situation. In this extreme situation the children (who may be adult by now) have either to submit to a process whereby they are institutionalized in the family setting[1]

---

[1] One has known many families in which parents function as unpaid mental nurses or psychiatrists. These parents prepare daily, weekly, monthly, and annual reports on their offspring. They often invoke the customary jargon of psychiatrists: 'He was very impulsive and uncooperative this morning, we telephoned his employers to explain but could not get him off to work – he probably needs more stelazine'. Or, 'He told his mother last night that he hated her, that he had

or to submit to periodic psychiatric hospitalization, which amounts to much the same thing. The only way out of this position is to die completely and completely to be reborn, if human circumstances permit, in a new, adequate identity.

Other people, however, can make do with nothing more than temporary partial deaths followed by phases of renewal. Such people can achieve their ends by momentary craziness, catching themselves up again before invalidation supervenes, or by lysergic acid diethylamide or mescaline or marijuana, or simply by getting drunk, or by listening to some music or seeing a picture which shatters their pre-established inner order and promotes or provokes an autonomous effort to piece themselves together again. All aesthetic experience consists in this sort of adventure. The first movement of the classical sonata pre-establishes an order with the statement of the subjects and then proceeds by a highly disciplined means to disintegrate this order in the development. The development, as is the case with all human development that transcends musculo-skeletal growth, is where one sweats it out in the turning moment of disintegration–reintegration. The recapitulation finally establishes the renewed first and second subjects.

What one should note here is the invention of a discipline for disintegration. For people who are being shattered to pieces psychiatry should provide the clue to the personal invention of such an essential discipline – but this is not what actually happens. Instead the patient encounters either ritually applied techniques of 'physical treatment' that are often a panic-stricken effort to blot out his intolerable experienced reality or, if he is marginally more fortunate, he encounters a literally fantastic complex of group meetings with every possible combination of nominally de-hierarchized staff and patients conjoined in their desperation to sort him out and knock him into any sort of shape but his own.

not yet been born, that he wanted to drag her guts out of her into the daylight, he was confused and had delusions and heard voices telling him he was bad, evil, bad . . . I'm sure he needs to come back into hospital.' Another father scored up the number of barbiturate pills his addicted son took per day, per week, and per year—each month this enigmatic sum would be duly posted in to the doctor. There are indeed many remedies for guilt.

The small but important minority of people entering mental hospitals who actually go mad (disintegrate) need psychiatrists and nurses who have sufficiently outgrown their fear, who have been at least relatively honest about their own madness, who have become capable of sanity by preferring it to normality. What was needed, I felt, in initiating a new type of psychiatric situation, was not techniques, or a programme, but the right people.

CHAPTER V

Villa 21 – An Experiment in Anti-Psychiatry

With the foregoing considerations in mind I undertook to run a ward in a large (2,000 bed) mental hospital just north-west of London on lines that would be bound to differ from the conventional ones. My experience of conventional psychiatric wards had been that these were places in which alienation, estrangement, and subtle violence were rife. Patients in such wards met with a massive reinforcement of the invalidation process that had commenced prior to their admission. It was in the admission ward that the ritual of initiation into the 'career' of being a mental patient was usually completed. It could perhaps, however, become the final exit from this process.

The inception of the unit in Villa 21 in January 1962 was brought about in an effort to satisfy three principal needs with which I was confronted in the actual situation in the mental hospital in which I worked.

First, there were practical organizational problems: I felt it to be unsatisfactory that adolescents who presented acting-out disturbances and also young schizophrenics[1] in their first acute breakdown were treated in wards in which the majority of patients were far advanced in a series of recurrent psychotic breakdowns. Such breakdowns acquire a limiting ritualistic

[1] In the following pages I shall use terms such as 'schizophrenic', 'patients', 'treatment' with implied inverted commas. I have already thrown, and shall later in this volume throw, considerable doubt on the validity of these labels, but for the moment I shall simply recognize that the labels are used and I shall employ this usage. I would also point out that, although I often use the present tense, I in fact departed from Villa 21 in April 1966.

character through repeated hospital admission. Sometimes young people would even go into long-stay or very disturbed wards. There seemed an obvious need for a separate unit with less ritual and less rigid role-structuring, where the patients could encounter themselves through their relationships with others and come to terms more successfully with their conflicts, rather than take the easy exit into narrowly sterotyped self-definition which is only too readily available to people in more conventional wards.

I felt too, somewhat uncertainly, that staff anxiety about adolescent sexual and aggressive acting-out might less readily result in disastrous blind repressive measures if this acting-out were more geographically localized within the total institution. I was, however, very aware of the possibility of the unit becoming to some extent a scapegoat into which 'badness' in the hospital would be projected, with consequent administrative conflict, rather than becoming a coping mechanism for the wider institution.

Secondly, there were research needs. In particular there was the need for a suitable working-situation for group and family-interactional research in schizophrenia and, more generally, in disturbed adolescence. Observations on such interaction had proved difficult in the hectic atmosphere of a general admission ward with its extreme heterogeneity of personal problems. Also there was the need for comparative data on interaction in families and in specialized therapeutic groups.

Thirdly, there was the need to establish a viable prototype for a small autonomous unit which could function in a large house in the community, outside the psychiatric institutional context. It was the author's belief that such small units might form the optimal therapeutic milieu for the sort of patients we had in mind, as they would allow a greater degree of freedom of movement out of the highly artificial staff and patient roles imposed on people by conventional psychiatry. But first of all it was necessary to explore the limits of change possible within the large mental hospital, to note the difficulties and contradictions that would arise, and to base future plans on such an assessment.

The insulin coma ward became available for the unit with the gradual cessation of insulin coma treatment. This ward comprised nineteen beds upstairs (a dormitory and four side-rooms) and downstairs accommodation including a sitting-room, dining-room, staff office and cloak-room, and two small rooms, one of which was used for small group meetings and the other as a quiet room. There were lavatories downstairs and lavatories and bath-room (one bath) upstairs. The main through corridor separated the staff office and the lavatories from the patients' living accommodation.

The patients were men aged between fifteen and the late twenties. Over two-thirds had been independently diagnosed as schizophrenic, the rest bore such labels as adolescent emotional crisis or personality disorder. At first we took in patients in these categories from other wards in the hospital, some of them with a history of several years of hospitalization. Gradually, over the first few months these patients moved on and we took in people in their first or second psychotic breakdown who had had relatively little experience of institutionalization.

Staff selection was made over a period of a year prior to the opening of the ward as a 'treatment unit'. This entailed many individual and group discussions. The selective process centred on the younger charge and staff nurses whose attitude to their work was less likely to be institutionally deformed and who seemed best able to tolerate the inevitable anxieties of group-therapeutic work. One charge nurse and one staff nurse were finally selected for each of the two day shifts. In addition there was to be a student nurse on each shift, but this staff member would have to change ward every two to four months to gain experience in other wards as part of his training programme.

A special request was made to the Nursing Office to minimize change of the night nurse, as this form of inconstancy has frequently been noted to disturb psychotic patients. A fulltime female occupational therapist for the ward was selected and one of the psychiatric social workers accepted her normal professional role in the unit along with her responsibilities for other wards.

85

Initially three doctors worked in the unit – each in a daily therapeutic group of between five and seven patients. At this stage community meetings (all the patients and all the staff) were held only twice a week. After some months, partly due to the felt need for more regular community meetings and partly because of a reorganization of the doctors' time-commitments, it was decided to hold daily community meetings from 9.45 to 10.15 a.m. followed by two 'doctors' groups' from 10.30 to 11.30 a.m. One of the doctors (the author) was then able to allocate most of his time to therapy and research in the unit (although his other work included the care of 120 long-stay patients and six to ten hours per week outpatient work). One other doctor, who was officially employed only on a part-time basis, in fact far exceeded her obligatory time-commitments: although she spent most of her time in the unit she also, together with another doctor, worked with about 200 long-stay and 'refractory' patients and held a weekly outpatient clinic. This situation reflected the general problem of gross staff shortage, but it was nevertheless possible to achieve a working minimum of psychiatrist time-commitment in the unit.

The original programme of the unit was deliberately a highly structured one, not unlike that of the 'classical' therapeutic community. This was not because I had any illusions about the limitations of such a model, but because it seemed strategically necessary to start off from a point that was not too 'far out'.

In the initial programme, groups were regarded as either 'scheduled' or 'spontaneous'.[1] Scheduled groups consisted of:

(a) *The daily community meeting* which ran from 9.45 to 10.15 or 10.30 a.m. (prior to 9.45 a.m. the doctors and social worker attended the divisional meeting of doctors on the male side of the hospital). This meeting, which was attended by all the patients and staff of the ward, was geared to communication about problems which affected the whole ward – usually disturbing acting-out on the part of an individual or sub-

---

[1] I feel compelled to remind any readers of my inverted commas and irony at this point.

group, or staff or patient grumbles, or practical arrangements for the work and recreational activities.

(b) The two more formal *therapeutic groups* in which half the patients met from 10.30 to 11.30 a.m. with one of the doctors and either the charge or staff nurse who constantly attended that particular group: the nature of these groups is described more fully later.

(c) *Work groups* – two groups which met from 2.00 to 4.30 p.m., each afternoon – one group with the occupational therapist, the other with a staff nurse; each group had its own project, the two longest-term projects in the first year being an interior decoration group and a toy-making group.

(d) *Staff group meetings* – the staff group met daily, briefly and informally, before and after the community meeting, and again often late in the afternoon; there was also a 'change-over' meeting once a week in which both nursing shifts met with the doctors and occupational therapist to discuss in particular unit policy matters for which cross-shift continuity was essential; once a week there was a full staff meeting for one hour, attended by the ward staff, the psychiatric social worker, and often a representative from the nursing administrative office and the head of the occupational therapy department.

'Spontaneous' groups formed at any time of the day or night around some particular issue – anything from discussion of a television programme to attempts to deal with disturbing acting-out on the part of some patient. A staff member would be 'in on' most of such groups, but the expectation was set up in the structuring of the unit that someone would communicate significant happenings in spontaneous groups to the community meeting.

In setting up the unit, I had one central conviction. This conviction, founded on repeated unhappy experiences in conventional wards, was that before we have any chance of understanding what goes on in patients we have to have at least some

elementary awareness about what goes on in the staff. We therefore aimed to explore in our day-to-day work the whole range of
preconceptions, prejudices, and fantasies that staff have about
each other and about the patients.

This is undoubtedly a major task. The psychiatric institution
throughout its history has found it necessary to defend itself
against the madness which it is supposed to contain – disturbance,
disintegration, violence, contamination. The staff defences, in so
far as they are erected against illusory rather than real dangers, I
shall term collectively *institutional irrationality*. What then, is the
reality of madness in the mental hospital and what is illusion?
What are the defining limits of institutional irrationality? In this
chapter I shall attempt at least to sketch in some of these limits.

It has long been recognized that a great deal of violent behaviour in mental patients is directly reactive to physical restraint.
If any member of the public were to be seized by several burly
men and thrust into a strait-jacket for reasons which were obscure
to him, and if his attempts to find an explanation were without
avail, his natural reaction would be to struggle. We are no longer
in the era of strait-jackets, and padded rooms are on the way out,
but it is not so long ago that the writer saw a patient, kicking and
screaming in a strait-jacket, carried by several policemen into the
observation ward: one had only to dismiss the policemen and
remove the strait-jacket dramatically to terminate the patient's
violent reactions.

Today many psychiatrists resort to 'chemical restraint' – seda-
tives and tranquillizers – and to electro-shock and bed-rest. The
effect of these apparently less drastic measures, however, is much
the same as the more drastic if they are used, as they often are,
without any reasonable explanation. The expectation set up when
a patient is given a large dose of tranquillizer is that there is
danger in him which must be controlled. Patients who are very
sensitive to such expectations often oblige by providing the
violence – at least until they are subdued by a larger dose of the
same 'treatment'. This is not to say that disturbed patients should
not sometimes be given tranquillizers, but simply that there

should be clarity in the doctor and in the patient about what is being done. There rarely is. The meaning of this situation is only too often lost in the quasi-medical mystique of 'illness' and 'treatment'. Why should one not, for instance, tell the patient: 'I'm giving you this stuff called Largactil to quieten you down a bit so that we can get on with other pressing things without feeling too anxious about what you are going to get up to next!'

One of the commonest staff fantasies in mental hospitals is that if patients are not coerced verbally or physically into getting out of bed at a certain hour in the morning they will stay in bed until they rot away. Behind this is anxiety over nonconformity with the staff's time-regulation and general control in their own lives. The patient is that frightening aspect of themselves that sometimes does not want to get out of bed in the morning and come to work. It is obviously true that if they succumbed to this temptation, they would lose their jobs. It is also true that young schizophrenic patients will eventually leave hospital and take jobs which they will have to attend punctually. But all this ignores the life-historical significance of the 'staying in bed problem'. In the past the patient has probably depended entirely on his mother to get him up in the morning. Shortly prior to his admission he has often rebelled against this forced dependence by what, for various reasons, is the only course available to him, namely staying in bed despite his mother's efforts to get him up. This 'withdrawal' is often one of the 'presenting symptoms' of schizophrenia.

In hospital one can repeat the family pattern, that is to say, gratify the patient's dependent needs by getting him up, but this is really getting up *for him*. Or one can take the 'risk' of leaving the decision to him in the hope that he will one day *get up himself*.

In fact, after many heated discussions of this issue in the unit and a great deal of policy difference between the nursing shifts, it was found that if the usual vigorous rousing procedures were abandoned and patients left to get up themselves, they invariably did rise, even if in some cases they would spent most of the day in bed for several weeks. No one rotted away after all and the gain in personal autonomy seemed worth while.

Staff at first and then patients would comment in the community meetings on the getting-up problem in terms of dependent needs, but the point was also brought home in more active ways. At one time all the occupants of a six-bed dormitory rebelled against the community meeting by staying in bed until after eleven o'clock. Frank, one of the charge nurses went upstairs to see what was going on. One of the patients left to go to the toilet and Frank seized the opportunity to take off his white coat[1] and climb into the vacant bed. The patient, on his return, appreciating the irony of the situation, had little option but to take the vacated 'staff role', put on the white coat, and get the others out of bed.

Another fantasy prevalent in the mental hospital concerns patient work. It is held implicitly, and sometimes stated, that if patients are not fully occupied in domestic ward jobs and the various occupational therapy projects, or helping in hospital maintenance departments, they will become 'withdrawn', 'institutionalized' 'chronic patients'. The bitter truth is that if they submissively carry out all these required tasks, they become what is implied by these labels anyhow. If one wishes to encounter the ultimate in withdrawn chronic institutionalization, one has only to visit one of the more 'active' and productive 'factories in a hospital' or 'industrial occupational therapy departments.' There is, relatively speaking, something remarkably healthy about the chronic schizophrenic, preoccupied with his inner world, spending the day hunched over the central heating fitting in a decrepit back ward. If he does not have the solution to the riddle of life, at least he has fewer illusions.

In the unit we had some desperate confrontations on this matter. Patients resisted conventional occupational therapy projects. We had begun to question the ancient myth that tells us that Satan makes work for idle hands, or 'work and play, don't

---

[1] Nurses in the unit occasionally wear their white coats not as uniforms but as protective clothing when joining in some messy job such as washing-up.

masturbate', but were not certain about where we went from there. Work projects would at least form a group, make a happy ward family. But perhaps people had come to the hospital to get away from 'happy families'. Or rather they had been sent to hospital to keep the family happy. We worked through a number of virile destructive jobs, knocking down an air-raid shelter, breaking up an aero engine: these jobs, some felt, would provide a 'safe outlet' for 'dangerous aggressive impulses'. These jobs, however, were done without enthusiasm and we soon began to realize their irrelevance to the real problems of anger. People had real reasons to be angry with real other people at home and in hospital (this was not entirely reducible to projection). The aero engine was an innocent party.

Our anxieties led us to put forward, consider, and then reject a number of other typical hospital projects of a ludicrously trivial nature, such as putting together the manufactured elements in (ironically) toy doctor's sets. Patients reacted contemptuously to these tasks and we came to share their feelings. Most of them were young men of at least average intelligence, well able to acknowledge the incongruity of the projects offered them. We visited local factories in an attempt to find more 'realistic' work for the patients on commission for the firm but nothing effective was achieved. In retrospect this was hardly surprising. We concluded that the only realistic jobs for the young people who came to us were jobs *outside* the hospital.

It was only after the first year of the unit's life that the staff, including the young female occupational therapist, were able to tolerate a situation in which no organized work project was presented to the community. Whatever project had been offered disintegrated after some weeks when patients 'skived off' to private activities elsewhere within and outside the hospital. Sanctions in the form of reduction of pocket money[1] did not affect the issue at all. What were we getting so anxious about, and what were we trying to do anyhow?

The occupational therapist, who had already abandoned her

[1] Up to 22s. 6d. per week allowance for patients who work in the hospital.

green uniform, found herself gravitating towards a role that seemed nearer to the nursing role. She even considered resigning and joining the staff as an assistant nurse. It was at this time that we became particularly aware of the fact of role diffusion, the breakdown of role boundaries, which was a necessary stage on the way to staff and patients defining themselves and their relationships with each other not on the basis of an imposed, abstract labelling system, reflecting a few technical or quasi-technical functions, but in terms of the personal reality of each member of the community.

There was a progressive blurring of role between nurses, doctor, occupational therapist, and patients. I have already examined some of the ambiguities surrounding the process of 'becoming a patient'. I shall now try to bring into focus a number of disturbing and apparently paradoxical questions: for example, can patients 'treat' other patients, and can they even treat staff? Can staff realize quite frankly and acknowledge in the ward community their own areas of incapacity and 'illness' and their need for 'treatment'? If they did, what would happen next and who would control it? Were not these categories 'illness' and 'treatment' themselves ultimately suspect.

It was at this point that the most radical departure from conventional psychiatric work was initiated. If the staff rejected prescribed ideas about their function, and if they did not quite know what to do next, why do anything? Why not withdraw from the whole field of hospital staff and patient expectation in terms of organizing patients into activity, supervising the ward domestic work, and generally 'treating patients'. The staff group decided to limit their function to controlling the drug cupboard as was legally required (some of the more 'overactive and impulsive' patients were on the tranquillizer, Largactil) and to dealing with ward administrative issues involving other hospital departments over the telephone.

A necessary prelude to this major policy change was explanation to the nursing office and other hospital departments. The kitchen staff for instance were informed that if the aluminium food containers were returned unwashed they should leave them until they were cleaned rather than telephone us complaining that the staff were not doing their job. If people wanted to eat they would have to clean the containers. These decisions were made quite clear to everyone in the community meetings.

Despite these explanations and the superficial acceptance of them, the events that followed were dramatic. In the first phase rubbish accumulated higher and higher in the corridors. Dining-room tables were covered with the previous days' unwashed plates. Signs of horror were evoked in visiting staff, in particular nursing officers on their twice-daily rounds. Patients decided their own leave periods, getting out of bed, attendance at meetings. Staff were anxious throughout, but particularly because no patients showed signs of organizing themselves to attend to these matters. A night nurse, who had previously worked as a day staff nurse in the unit, finally became so exasperated that he officially reported the filthy state of the ward to the night superintendent. The chief male nurse was informed and nursing officers visited the ward duly to express their disgust at the state of affairs. The anger of the night nurse we acknowledged as to some extent our fault: communication between day and night shifts was clearly inadequate (it had only been with considerable difficulty that we had been able to initiate regular cross-shift meetings between the two day shifts – an arrangement that was later replaced by a system in which most staff worked cross-shift).

External administrative pressure on the ward staff rapidly mounted. The patients were divided in their response. Some began to demand more nurse and doctor attention. Those less urgently dependent expressed some dissatisfaction but at the same time made it clear that they appreciated the more authentic elements in the policy change.

Subsequent events must be seen in relation to the problem of doctor-centredness in mental hospital ward administration. In conventional wards all but the most trivial decisions have to be either made by, or blessed by, the doctor. The doctor is invested, and sometimes invests himself, with magical powers of understanding and curing. Whether the formal training of psychiatrists includes qualifications in magical omnipotence is perhaps uncertain, but the image is reinforced and perpetuated in many ways. The same person who is supposed to have a psychotherapeutic relationship with patients assumes a general practitioner role in relation to their bodily ailments. Not only that, but psychiatrists attend the staff sick bay and medically care for nurses with whom they work. The resulting confusion of controlled frustration and wholesale gratification can well be imagined.

If the white coat and stethoscope provide one means by which the psychiatrist defends himself from patients, that is to say from his own projected disturbance, the printed form is another. Doctors have accepted, only too readily in many cases, a mass of legal and administrative responsibilities which keep them from getting near their patients but which, to a far greater extent than is commonly admitted, could be left to efficient, suitably trained non-medical administrators. As things stand, however, the doctor visiting the ward includes a pile of official forms and certificates in his (often unwanted) armamentarium and these forms structure his relationships with staff and patients before anything else he does or they do has any effect.

In addition to this medical, legal, and administrative pre-structuring of the psychiatrist's role, there are occasionally more realistic factors that lead to his assumption of the central position in the ward, namely training and experience in psycho-therapeutic skills and small group sociology. These skills, however, are by no means universal among psychiatrists and are conspicuously minimized in, or absent from, most training courses for diplomas in psychiatry. Some members of selection committees are prejudiced against formal psycho-analytic training, and in any case such training is beyond the means of most young married psychiatrists – who get no income tax relief on what amounts to a yearly cost of about £500 for four or five years.

These and other considerations mean that staff and patients in the ward expect the doctor to take a leader role. In the staff groups the level of dependency on the doctor is not much different from that in the staff-patient groups. The problem for nurses is to change their position from one in which they mediate the doctor-for-the-patient and the patient-for-the-doctor to one in which they frankly and 'legitimately' involve themselves in relationships without the mediating or mediated 'third'. In the mental hospital, each transaction between persons has either, against all the odds, to struggle free of pseudo-medical deformation or be reduced to a purely formal, inauthentic manoeuvre. This shift of position is fantastically difficult. After three years of work centred largely on this issue we have barely shifted at all in the unit – but we have shifted a little.

It was during the 'experimental' phase of staff withdrawal that the staff group was able to make some advance. The author was away on holiday in Eastern Europe for a month. Official pressure on the unit to introduce conventional controls was at its peak. Anxiety among the staff was considerable and there was an added factor of conflict between the two shifts (7 a.m. to 2 p.m. and 2 p.m. to 9 p.m.) of nurses. Much of the latter conflict was based on the mistaken attribution of certain intentions to the doctor. The suggestion that staff should withdraw from their supervisory, directive role, informing the patients how this would happen, was in fact generated by one shift of nurses. This was gently confirmed by the doctor (the author) and was seemingly accepted with only a few, unimportant reservations by the whole staff group. Two nurses on the other shift, however, fostered an unexpressed antagonism to the change. Because of earlier happenings in the unit which had led to the idea among hospital staff that the unit doctor had new, 'ultra-permissive' ideas, the staff decision was regarded as the 'doctor's policy' – it might be pretty crazy but if it originated in the mind of a senior doctor it was unquestionable.

The advance made by the staff group was frankly to recognize their anxiety as intolerable and, in the doctor's absence, to arrive at a 'group decision' to re-impose some staff controls on what went on in the ward. It was decided to supervise eating and cleaning arrangements and to insist on attendance at community meetings and adherence to the rule that weekend leave was only granted from Saturday morning (after the community meeting) to Sunday night. It was decided that persistent offenders against these rules would have to choose between conforming to them or discharge from the unit. On my return I lent my confirmation to these decisions and in fact two patients were shortly discharged (in both cases this confrontation with a group reality led to favourable consequences).

At bottom the problem is one of distinguishing between authentic and inauthentic authority. The actual practice of a great deal of psychiatry in this country, whatever progressive mantle it may don, aims at enforcing conformism to the rigid, stereo-typed dictates of authority persons. Such persons by refraction condense on to the patient various social expectations and hidden injunctions as to who and what he may be. These expectations and injunctions are often quite alien to the individual needs and individual reality of the patient. The authority of the authority person is granted him by arbitrary social definition rather than on the basis of any real expertise he may possess. If staff have the courage to shift themselves from this false position they may discover real sources of authority in themselves. They may also discover such sources in the others who are defined as their patients. This begins to get disturbing – particularly when the patients sometimes happen to be those who are clinically the most psychotic in the ward. One of the most memorable group meetings in the unit was dominated by an extremely fragmented patient who was just beginning a lengthy project of reintegration. All the staff and patients were lulled into a fascinated somnolence by his account of a 'bizarre', imaginary world tour. We became a sort of collective infant at the breast of the mother-narrator. I made a formal comment in these terms but interpretation was not necessary. At a certain point indicated by the narrator everyone snapped out of the phantasy awareness to find themselves on a more integrated level of group reality. And there was no doubt about who had led them there.

Perhaps the most central characteristic of authentic leadership is the relinquishing of the impulse to dominate others. Domination here means controlling the behaviour of the others where their behaviour represents for the leader projected aspects of his own experience. By domination of the other the leader produces for himself the illusion that his own internal organization is more and more perfectly ordered. The mythical prototype of the inauthentic leader is William Blake's Urizen, the man of the horizon, of limits, control, order, imposed because of terror of *his own* free field of possibilities. Some leaders dare to see the world with clear eyes, others prefer to envision it through their fundament. The Nazi extermination camps were one product of this Dream of Perfection. The mental hospital, along with many other institutions in our society, is another. In the camp bodily existences were systematically annihilated, each body containing, in terms of the illusion, the projected badness, sexual anomaly, meanness of the camp officials and the society they represented. This murder was always ritual murder aimed at the purification of the murderer and, as it was essentially a manner of evading guilt, how can one suppose that the murderers should feel guilty *because* of it? In the mental hospital bodies are assiduously cared for but individual personalities are murdered. The model system for the conventional mental nurse and psychiatrist is the delightfully landscaped cabbage patch. As cabbages exist comfortably enough, at least until they go into the soup, many patients choose to collude with the illusions of their keepers, and this interplay of illusion and collusion is the basic social phantasy-system upon which the structure of the mental hospital is erected. It is plainly a totally alienated structure.

Although staff in the unit have been able to discover in themselves some elements of authentic leadership, the situation in which they function is replete with contradictions. Most of the nurses live in hospital accommodation (the nurses' home or separate houses on the hospital estate). The student nurses and sometimes staff nurses have to leave to work in other wards; all nurses are dependent on the central nursing administration for promotion. Outside the unit they are subjected to very strong direct social and indirect financial pressures to conform and this inevitably becomes a pressure to conform inside the unit. The staff social club and village pubs foster this insinuated indoctrination. But conformism in this context means a reversion to the prevalent primitive, ritualized nursing attitudes that run counter to the culture that has developed in the unit. This means that nurses must choose between submission to external pressures, on the one hand, and adherence to the unit principles, on the other. Until they do choose, their existence in the unit is inevitably painfully confused. The extent to which the staff group in the unit can help them is limited by the reality of the dilemma and the necessity for commitment one way or the other.

We should reflect a moment here on the magnitude of the anxieties involved. For the unit nurses these issues quite literally went 'right home' – to their families involved in the social life and promotion struggle of the hospital as a whole. When they refused to quit their ideological ground they faced ridicule, sometimes amounting to attributions, half behind their backs, of madness. For some senior nurses outside the unit, on the other hand, the demand to re-establish controls and 'tidy up' things assumed the dimensions of a desperate struggle between life and death forces, sanity and madness. They felt intensely threatened by all the things in the unit that infringed the staff-patient dividing line, e.g. patients calling staff by their first names, staff and patients having tea together, the suggestion that ex-patients be employed as nurses (since there was an acute shortage of nurses, and since we felt that their personal qualities and experience of breakdown and recovery in the unit would make them particularly useful in the staff group). These developments and many others challenged their conceptions of themselves as sane in relation to the mad patients. The gravity of these anxieties was sometimes masked by the ludicrously trivial nature of incidents that lead to crises. On one occasion, for instance, a nursing officer on his rounds sent in a report criticizing ward staff for lack of supervision when he observed a patient pouring milk into his tea from a bottle rather than use the thoughtfully provided milk-jug in the cupboard. When one of the staff commented that he often did this himself at home the situation was not helped.

Nowhere were anxieties more evident than in the highly significant distortions of the hospital communication process. Reports are submitted to the nursing office by the nurse in charge of the unit at the end of each shift. Sometimes these reports travel via the night nursing superintendent to the day shift of nursing administrators. At each change of hands the reports are edited, 'significant' happenings in each ward being selected for presentation in a final version to the daily meeting of doctors, social workers, and nursing officers on the division.[1] A typical incident processed by this communication system was the following: a young man in the unit had a girl-friend in a female ward; one night she became hysterically upset about an issue connected with her ward and treatment, and he and a friend attempted to console her and help her back to her ward; she noisily resisted these attempts and a member of the portering staff who witnessed the incident called a nurse who took her back to her ward. The porter informed the night nursing superintendent, who informed the unit and reported to the day nursing administration, who reported finally to the divisional meeting. The final version was that two male patients from the unit had attacked a female patient and, it was implied, were attempting to carry her off for sexual purposes. The fantasy existing in the minds of many staff outside the unit is that rape, sexual orgies, and murder are daily occurrences in the unit – and this is not entirely rhetorical exaggeration on my part. In fact, during the last two years there was no significant injury produced by patient violence in the unit and no pregnancy in young female patients who frequently visited boyfriends in the unit and went out with them.

Crises arise and then subside but they cannot indefinitely be 'tidied over'. The mental hospital as a social system defines itself by certain limits within which change is possible, but beyond which one cannot venture without threatening the stability of the

[1] The whole hospital of 2,100 patients was divided into three more or less self-contained divisions each led by a consultant psychiatrist.

whole structure. This structure as it has developed historically has acquired institutional sclerosis. This fact is proved repeatedly by the experience of the incipient disintegration in the whole institutional world of relationship and non-relationship when one pushes out rather hard against the limits of the structure.

To sum up on the present state of development of the unit, I think the following things have to be said. During the four years of the unit's life we have progressively and successfully eliminated many destructive aspects of psychiatric institutional life. We have eliminated formal hierarchization to a point beyond which no similar experiment in the literature of the subject has gone – at least with diagnosed schizophrenic patients. In doing this we have rid ourselves of the rigid grading of inmates into patients and staff (the staff being in turn sub-graded into an indefinitely extensible hierarchy of student nurse, assistant nurse, staff nurse, charge nurse or sister, nursing officer, ward doctor, various ranks of administrator, consultants, etc).

A certain basic materiality in the situation remains. Staff are paid to be there, patients are not. Staff are paid according to their official role and rank. It is clear, however, that an 'untrained' assistant nurse or a patient may manifest more healing potential than a given high-ranking staff member. There are many things in the existing forms of training for mental nurses and psychiatrists that simply obscure the trainee's vision of the realities in his field of work. Such training involves a great deal of indoctrination into the tactics of staff defence against patients. The old hands recall their years of 'experience' and protest against grandmother being taught how to suck eggs. But, of course, years in a mental hospital do not necessarily imply any experience at all, they may amount quite simply to time-serving. As one 'junior' staff member pointed out, if grandmother has not yet learned how to suck eggs she may have to be taught.

We have refused to isolate the hospitalized member of a family as 'the ill one' and have attempted in many cases to delineate his role, concretely as well as theoretically, as that of the victim, the one who sacrifices his personal autonomous existence so that those others of his family-world may live, relatively free of guilt. We have witnessed and confirmed in our encounter with him his realization, however partial and distorted, of the Christ-archetype. Without elevating him to the cheaply won status of the 'Schizophrenic as Culture-Hero' we have at least partially eliminated the distance between him ('the lunatic') and us ('the staff'), the representatives of the sane society, and have found a way together with him of treasuring what is called his madness, although this has been not without enormous envy and a perpetual edging back on the part of the staff.

We have also, with very little organizational support, helped him to make reasonable arrangements for his independent life when he leaves the mental hospital. These arrangements have very often fallen through and the patient has subsequently had to make use of the unit, perhaps as a place to stay for a weekend or sometimes for a few weeks. But this, for reasons which I shall make explicit, has seemed to us to be due to circumstances that are beyond our immediate control and should be the business of the community to organize – in terms which are both legally implied (Mental Health Act, 1959) and supported by 'moral conviction'. For want of such community organization we have arranged through personal contact for some discharged patients to live with reliable people (i.e. non-mystifying, minimally anxious people) in houses in the community in small groups. These projects (which will be described in future publications) present the best and most creative alternative to the stultifying or even untenable position that the patient gets into in his family home and in the institution.

In the staff group discussions and also in discussions with visitors to the unit we have learnt more about the distinction between the purified formal group-analytic situation and a real community. In the group-analytic situation there is a rigorous avoidance of certain group experiences that in the community we would regard as essential. This avoidance is conducted in the name of a sort of demystification – that is to say people (the analytic subjects) are demystified in terms of their phantastic hopes of gratification from the therapist as parent-figure. But on the other hand in the unit there were some of us, including the author, who felt that in the actual group atmosphere there was a terrible lack, something missing from the total world of our experience, that could not be reduced to interpretation of the 'group-transference'. What I hope we have learned to avoid doing is to see this lack in terms of some hypothetical 'schizophrenic' system of needs. In so far as this can be put in the language of need, it is the needs of every one of us that are involved and that must be inspected.

At one stage, and this was in fact an oft-repeated motif, the view was expressed in the community meetings that the principal difference between staff and patients was that staff were able to leave the unit at the end of their duty period and go home to their wives or girl-friends and have sexual relations: the patients on the other hand never left the unit, apart from, in some cases, having weekends home with their parents, and lived in a situation of total sexual frustration except for occasional masturbation in the toilet. Beyond the literal aspect of this 'sex-talk' however, was a more basic notion of failure. The word 'fucking' meant for people in the unit nothing more or less than real contact between people. It meant meeting, encounter, and this extension beyond the literal meaning was repeatedly made clear in the community meetings. On walking into a community meeting one has encountered sometimes, in the early stages, a staff group which, sitting like stuffed zoological specimens, certainly possessed a classificatory significance but was most uncertain about what was their human reality in relation to that of 'their patients'. Staff were in fact very carefully selected from among the existing nurses in the hospital and these were the best people that could be found – but their difficulties, as I have indicated, were immense.

This aptly expresses the stage which the unit reached currently. Staff can only proceed into the reality of what the unit community is at the price of sacrificing their livelihoods or at least placing them in an uncertain degree of jeopardy. We have been nudging into that most threatening borderland between staff and patients, sanity and madness. When we suggested that patients discharged from the unit might in fact be the best nurses in at least one aspect of nursing, the official response was far from promising. In fact the possibility of our employing such people was ruled out in principle. Among the arguments preferred was above all else the view that such people could not be sufficiently 'stable' to cope with the 'stresses' of mental nursing. Although I have put stresses in inverted commas these stresses are real enough but they are not what conventionally minded nurses and doctors seem to think they are. It is not only a matter of conflict between so many calculable masses of brawn and it is certainly not a matter of the capacity of nurses to posit as such and then classify patients, that is to say to order them according to some metaphysically violent, if not physically violent, schema. The real difficulty for staff is to confront themselves, to confront their own problems, disturbances, madness. Each one has to risk meeting the lunatic in himself. The conventional equilibrium established by the externalization of the violence of psychiatrists and nurses (who act on behalf of 'the public') into patients will no longer pass uncriticized because it is unnoticed. It has produced the major social problem of the mental hospital by working a subtle and complex collusion with the family of the patient and, through the family, with the whole of mental health officialdom.

Today younger psychiatrists and nurses are beginning to resent the role, which is forced upon them, of being some sort of policemen for the rest of society. But of such young people very few have in fact learned thoroughly enough the lesson of self-criticism. The usual way out is through some half-compromising adjustment to social needs. Psycho-analytic training introduces an element of rigour but this is hardly enough to meet the demands of the situation, which are indeed extreme.

Mental hospitals were invented to 'look after' or (in rasher moments) to 'cure' sick persons. If the 'sickness' is called in question, and if the isolation of one patient–person from the more truly sick family system is shown to be a fallacy, then we are in an area of most radical questioning indeed.

The 'experiment' of the unit has had one quite certain 'result' and one certain 'conclusion'. The result is the establishment of the limits of institutional change, and these limits are found to be very closely drawn indeed – even in a progressive mental hospital. The conclusion is that if such a unit is to develop further, the development must take place outside the confines of the larger institution – which has been pushed physically outside the community, the matrix of family-worlds, where its real problems arise and where their answer lies. Specifically, staff who work in the unit must be liberated from the hierarchized, paternalistic system of domination by categorization. The unit must ultimately become a place to which people choose to come in order to escape, with authentic guidance, the inexorable process of invalidation that grinds on 'outside'. It must become this rather than a place by means of which 'the others' deviously rid themselves of their own scarcely perceived violence by a medically certified human sacrifice to the gods of a society that seems determined to sink and drown in the mud of its illusions.

We have had many pipe-dreams about the ideal psychiatric, or rather anti-psychiatric, community, but I believe we have now, by a process of demystification, sufficiently delineated the true nature of psychiatric madness and sufficiently worked out our practical needs to take a step forward.

And a step forward means ultimately a step out of the mental hospital into the community.

CHAPTER VI

Furthermore

Geoffrey H, who had recently graduated at Cambridge, came to visit my mental hospital. After some hours he found his way to the patients' social club in which patients from all wards in the hospital congregate for organized games and dancing. Inevitably a long-stay patient approached him, and then asked the remarkable question 'Hello, are you here?' The significance of this question resides in the patients' perception of the difference between staff and patients. Patients are 'here', inside; staff are not here: they come and go but, essentially, even if they live on the hospital estate and spend most of their spare time in the staff social club, they are outsiders. One savours this question with its implicit violence to ordinary meaning: 'are you here?' One reflects on the peculiar dialectic between 'here' and 'there'. The one who is here is not all there. Reciprocally the one who is not here is one who is there, that is to say not here, that is to say non-existent in the present actual circumstances. Geoffrey told me of his impressions of a mental hospital in these terms: solid but amorphous lumps of patients drifting around the grounds, gesturing, gesticulating, reviling, appealing – to thin air; shadowy imprints of staff engaged, if one may use so highly concrete a term, in jocular interaction or serious concerned discussion with patients and their fellow-staff: this man slaps another on his back but the back is not there, nor is the hand.

If the reification of persons, the highly convenient conversion of people into the things that surround them or oppose them, is carried beyond a certain critical point, we find that all that is left is an array of infinitely perfectible objects and human absences. A chief male nurse I spoke to recently at another hospital was concerned with the 'upgrading' of his wards. In pursuing this theme I discovered that the human contents of the wards and what they did with each other were far from the centrum of his anxiety. He was bothered about beds, the spacing of beds, the arrangement of coverlets, the quality of the food (his ideal, reasonably enough, was well-fried lamb chops, Worcester sauce, and chips) but, above all, he was worried about the condition of the toilets. This man who had achieved an ideal view of the world through the fundament, a thorough, systematically purged excremental vision, arranged for chromium-plated, centrally-heated lavatory pans to be inserted into one of the most congested long-stay wards. Outside the privy were angulated mirrors so that people using the convenience could see themselves and in particular the state of their trouser-flies through the eyes of a perfectly non-human Other.

This chief male nurse, however, was in no less fortunate a position than others who are implicated in the ambiguous hierarchy of the psychiatric division of the National Health Service. Compulsive orderliness is the key-word that must never be used in vain. The superintendent of another mental hospital with a very impressive discharge rate for schizophrenic patients told me recently that he gave all newly admitted schizophrenics ten to twenty routine electro-shocks because if he did not do this, his nursing staff would not only be unable to cope with the disturbed behaviour but above all would lose faith in their capacity to assist in the curing of patients. He had achieved by this means very good figures for early discharge and less frequent re-admission (what actually happened to his patients during and between admissions was quite simply an irrelevant and even, possibly, untidy issue). But this man could not compare with the medical superintendent, in another Commonwealth country, who came to his hospital in pyjamas and dressing gown before 8.0 a.m. each morning to administer electro-convulsive therapy to thirty or forty patients to get his day off to a good start. In fact, he even once returned from a holiday in Sweden to give twenty quick shocks to selected patients before he could fly back to resume his vacation with a clear conscience. Nor again has this chief male nurse, who appeals to the doctors for patients to be 'attacked' (his term) with treatment, anything in his experience to compare with the psychiatrist who will prescribe with a flourish of his pen a second, third, or even fourth leucotomy (brain-slicing) operation to rid his patient of the disease he perceives him to have. Some psychiatrists possess juvenile shock-boxes with miniature electrodes, and in the United States some have even performed leucotomy operations on babies who cry too much – or too little. The need for uniformity would seem to be limitless were it not for the remarkable fact that 'advanced' (or neolithic) psychiatry can produce even a uniform non-uniformity right up to the limit of the nth meta-game.

I suppose that the basic difficulty is to be found in the idea of 'curing' patients. Curing is so ambiguous a term; one may cure bacon, hides, rubber, or patients. Curing usually implies the chemical treatment of raw materials so that they may taste better, be more useful, or last longer. Curing is essentially a mechanistic perversion of medical ideals that is quite opposite in many ways to the authentic tradition of healing.

In psychiatry the fetishism of the Cure has had gravely destructive consequences. Papers are published in the medical press claiming good results with various treatments that enjoy a brief fashionable success. Psychiatrists announce on television that schizophrenic episodes can be cured in so many weeks, but the criteria of improvement remain highly obscure. For some workers the mere fact of discharge of the patient from hospital or his non-readmission within a year of discharge would seem to indicate at least a degree of cure. Or again his capacity to hold a job while he is out of hospital. Or a change in the patient such that the psychiatrist no longer detects in him his former 'symptoms'. I have tried to indicate in earlier chapters that so-called symptoms are usually intelligible forms of behaviour and I am afraid that the simple suppression of symptoms with drugs and shock often, in fact, produces a situation of lessened intelligibility and of lessened vitality in the inner life of the patient.

Curing is concerned with making the patient more acceptable to others so that the others (including the doctors and nurses) become less anxious about him, and with making him express less distress. Healing on the other hand is concerned with helping people become whole when to a varying extent they have gone to pieces. For some people at certain times in certain life-situations going to pieces may be necessary as a pre-condition for a process of renewal. Also distress and anguish may be necessary for personal growth. Premature interference by psychiatric treatment may arrest or distort these processes. It is to my mind indefensible to resort to economic arguments in terms of reducing hospital beds to justify this form of therapeutic ruthlessness. 'Schizophrenia' involves the whole lives of persons, it is not an 'attack' or 'dose' of something noxious. Our psychiatric task is first to allow and second to help the patient remain alive as a person throughout the process of destructuring and then restructuring of his inner world.

We have witnessed people, in a situation of non-interference, go into a progressive disintegration over weeks or months and then gradually come together again. We have also witnessed the destructiveness of unwisely administered physical treatments and of bureaucratic interference, for example, the enforced transfer of disturbed patients from open to closed wards at critical moments when continuity of the human environment is essential. Such disruptive happenings have often led to the patient becoming arrested on a certain 'level of regression'. While the patient is so fixed, efforts are then made to socialize him on that level, to produce a maximal non-disturbing conformity.

The sort of thing of which I found myself continually aware in Villa 21 is the startling *reality* of young schizophrenic patients. To proceed from some formal committee meeting to a group in the ward is to pass from a world in which the people concerned are totally estranged from their own systems of phantasy and inner reality, a world of reduced reality, to a world full of surprises, full of the shock of coming to life. Few of the people in the Villa had any significant organized talent but there was a sort of diffused fragmentary genius, perhaps something more between people than in them.

One young man created a disturbance in the hospital church. He had been obsessed for two years with the meaning of the sin against the Holy Spirit and one day decided to carry his investigation into what seemed to be the most obvious place. This bearded, wild-looking young man concealed himself behind the altar and when the congregation were duly settled down to the routine of worship he leaped out of his concealment with a terrorized blood-curdling yell. What might have been a rare spiritual occasion ended with his being escorted back to his ward, and to bed, by a couple of large male nurses. Or again David – who went to a football match. I asked David the next day if he went alone or in company: 'Oh no, I went by myself, with some friends'. Or Henry – who had had visions of the mysterious union of red and white roses and who had thought that time had stood still and that then the hands of clocks had started moving backwards until he found himself drowning in prehistoric slime. This perfect sixteen-year-old Dostoevskian idiot told a nurse, 'I never mind who ridicules me as long as a child never laughs at me.' I remember thinking once that schizophrenics were the strangled poets of our age. Perhaps it is about time that we, who would be healers, took our hands off their throats.

I have mentioned these instances of what goes on in mental hospitals to illustrate a problem that faces us regarding future developments. At present a great deal of planning of the psychiatric services is being undertaken. This planning is based on statistics (often challenged) regarding, for instance, the duration of patients' stay in hospital and the shift of treatment from large mental hospitals to small units in general hospitals. What is missing is some concrete grasp of the problem, some insight into what actually goes on in people. For instance, in the case of young schizophrenic patients, treatment in general hospital units would tend merely to reinforce the medical model with its inevitable mystification and invalidation of the patient: 'You can't really feel that way, you're just sick.' Also the proximity to more highly ritualized nursing attitudes must make the job of the nurse who does not wish to seek refuge in ritual more difficult.

On the other hand, there is the difficulty of providing officially approved forms of validation of the work that is done in a unit such as I have described in this book. Any tendency to get patients working, to get them out of hospital, and to keep them out as long as possible – and by any means – for the sake of keeping them out must run counter to one's efforts to understand what goes on. One needs time to understand, and patients certainly need time to learn to live with the fruits of understanding.

There is so far no methodology accepted by official sources of power and sponsors of medical publications by which one simply, but painstakingly and with a maximum of clarity, describes and evaluates the transformations in the experience and behaviour of a person or of a group. The demand is always for quantification, however spurious, misleading, or irrelevant. I would hold – and have given my reasons in the Introduction – that the nature of events such as I have described here cannot be forced into this false framework.

The first need is for a situation of greater autonomy in which staff who are prepared, in both the active and the passive sense, can continue this work. I have presented some of the difficulties of working within a traditional context. I do not think that the answer lies simply in geographical separation from a more conventional hospital environment – in fact, this is by no means essential. What is needed, however, is a sufficient degree of independence, since it is only on this basis that patients, with our assistance,[1] can renew themselves into a state of greater wholeness and therefore autonomy.

I have dealt with problems of autonomy by certain necessarily artificial means, for instance by having two sorts of nurse. On the

[1] Or, of course, 'we', with 'their' assistance.

one hand, conventionally trained nurses who, apart from their courage and integrity, qualified for the unit by possessing a highly developed instinctive awareness of the exigencies of bodily confrontation. These were sometimes people with a working-class Glasgow or Liverpool background who had learned from their earliest years how to handle aggression; how not to interfere prematurely in panic, but also how, at the right moment, to restrain someone in acute disturbance without hurting him. On the other hand, I introduced as social therapists (paid as Nursing Assistants) sensitive young people often with a university background (and often thought by regular staff to be a bit mad if not downright vicious) who could, without having to worry about a future in nursing, allow themselves to get close to the experience of disintegrated patients. If, however, we aim to achieve a state of wholeness in people, this sort of parcelling out of subtle roles cannot be desirable.

I believe that people who go into this work with a deliberate abandoning of most of the conventional staff defences are courageous pioneers. Society is perhaps only just ready to accept and even support such an innovation, but there are portents that this is so. We are no longer at a time when a simplistic common sense seems adequate to the contorted paradoxes of a man's inner voyage. I shall leave the reader to ponder the thick irony of Pascal: 'too much light darkens the mind'.[1]

---

[1] Later changed by an unusual failure of nerve to 'too much light dazzles the mind' (Brunschvicg's edition of the *Pensées et opuscules*, p. 353 note 6).

APPENDIX

The Question of Results
An Ironic Addendum

When the attempt is made to assess 'results' in a project such as Villa 21, there are two courses that may be followed. The first, which is the conventional one, ends up with a series of propositions expressing quantitative relations that are impressive in their statistical work-out but either meaningless or misleading in terms of what has actually happened to the persons concerned. The second course is to attempt a phenomenological description of the changes in the inner- and outer-world complexes of these persons, comparing these changes with certain possible changes that have previously been established as desirable or undesirable. The important point about this latter course is that the concern is with the actual experiences of actual persons and with individual fields of possibility.

The phenomenological approach does not mean that a level of generalization cannot be attained, but simply that it is necessary to commence with the concrete particular before proceeding to the abstract general. This approach, however, does not meet with general approval in most scientific and medical journals (cf. my remarks in the Introduction). Many research authorities in the human sciences seem to be victim to obsessional needs to reduce the reality of transactions between persons to massified abstractions that conceal far more than they reveal.

Despite this, there are, I believe, at least strategic reasons for looking at the work in terms of one of the less objectionable psychiatric criteria of 'improvement', namely the tendency of patients not to be re-admitted within one year of their discharge from hospital. For this reason I have included in this appendix a paper on the results of family-orientated therapy with schizophrenics written together with Dr A. Esterson and Dr R. D. Laing. I would point out, however, that these results refer[1] to a consecutive series of schizophrenic patients admitted in 1962. They do not reflect the overall picture in Villa 21. This is partly because up to one-third of patients in the unit at any time had non-schizophrenic diagnoses, most commonly 'adolescent emotional disturbance' or 'acting-out disorder'. Also, over the last two years discharged patients have been actively encouraged to avoid invalidatory crises outside by seeking informal readmission to the unit, often only for a day or two.

RESULTS OF FAMILY-ORIENTATED THERAPY WITH HOSPITALIZED SCHIZOPHRENICS

This is a report on the results of conjoint family and milieu therapy with hospitalized schizophrenics at two mental hospitals in the greater London area. During the past ten years the internal family milieu of schizophrenics has been intensively studied by workers in the United States (e.g. Bateson *et al.*, 1956; Lidz *et al.*, 1958; Wynne *et al.*, 1958), and by ourselves (Laing and Esterson, 1964). These studies, which have shown how frequently the person diagnosed as schizophrenic is part of a network of extremely disturbed and disturbing patterns of communication, have important implications for prevention, treatment, and after-care.

As a result both of this work, and of the work of psychotherapists with experience of prolonged relationships with schizophrenics, increasing doubt has been cast on the view that schizophrenia is a medical syndrome or entity in any sense

---

[1] As far as the male population in the sample is concerned – the female patients were not in Villa 21 but were in fact from another hospital.

employed currently in ordinary medical practice. This work has also rationalized a form of therapy that does not focus on the individual patient but on the group or system of communications of which he is part, whether within his family or within the mental hospital.

Principles of Method

Details of our method of family and group study and treatment of the person diagnosed schizophrenic will be described in subsequent publications.

Very briefly the principles we have followed are:

1. A systematic clarification and undoing of patterns of communication that we take to be 'schizogenic' within the family.
2. A similar clarification and undoing of such patterns of communication between patients and between staff and patients.
3. Continuity of personnel working with the family during and after the patient's stay in hospital.
4. None of the so-called shock treatments were used, nor was leucotomy. Patients received comparatively small doses of tranquillizers. For instance no male patient received more than the equivalent of 300 mgms. of chlorpromazine and 25 per cent of patients received no tranquillizers at all. Less than 50 per cent of the women and 15 per cent of the men received tranquillizers during the follow-up period.

A schizophrenic who is admitted to hospital is handicapped to a greater or lesser degree in his ability to live under ordinary social conditions. It is necessary to provide a social setting that takes this into account. We therefore reorganized the wards under our care to create a human context in which those transactions that our studies have shown are liable to precipitate psychotic behaviour were avoided as far as possible. In this context each patient was ensured of a relationship with at least one other person significant to him. This relationship was as consistent and reliable as we could achieve.

To this end we trained a team of social therapists selected from the nursing staff – a social therapist being any person who sets out to establish with the patient a consistent relationship of trust. We also used patients as social therapists.

The social therapist must be ready to use almost any situation to establish a relationship with a patient. He must be frank and honest at all times and be prepared to discuss honestly any issue no matter how personal to himself, or be straightforward in admitting his anxiety if he finds it impossible to discuss anything. Such readiness, whether in private or in a group, is crucial we believe to undoing the mystifying patterns of communication that surround the patient.

Selection

Our series consists of 42 patients, 20 men and 22 women, between the ages of fifteen and thirty-five, drawn from two mental hospitals in the London area. Patients were selected from consecutive schizophrenic admissions to hospital according to the following criteria, which were the same for both men and women:

1. They had been diagnosed as schizophrenic[1] by at least two senior psychiatrists not members of our therapeutic team, and were regarded as such by the staff.
2. They were not, and had not been, subjected to any organic condition (e.g. brain injury, epilepsy) that might have affected those functions regarded as disturbed in schizophrenics.
3. They were not of obviously subnormal intelligence.
4. They had not been subjected to brain surgery of any kind.
5. Nor had they received more than fifty electro-shocks in the year before the treatment began and not more than one hundred and fifty in all.
6. As for the family, at least one parent should be alive and available for interview. Patients could be with or without brothers

[1] The problem of the diagnosis, which of course enters into every report on schizophrenia, is extremely difficult, there being no generally agreed criteria or standards of reliability, regional, national or international. For a discussion of this question, see Kreitman (1961) and Laing and Esterson (1964).

or sisters, married or single, and with or without children. They could be living with their families or on their own. No patient or family refused to co-operate. Only one woman who met the other criteria was rejected because her parents not only lived too far away (in Scotland) but also because they were too infirm to travel. She was transferred to a hospital near them in accordance with administrative custom. Two of our patients were initially hospitalized in other parts of the country and had been transferred to our hospitals in order to be near their families. This was standard administrative procedure and was not the consequence of our research. Only one man who met our other criteria was rejected because both parents were dead. Presumably the low average age of our patients accounts for the ease with which this criterion was met.

The patients selected were otherwise clinically homogeneous with the schizophrenic intake to the two hospitals.[1]

Results
Our results are as follows.

All patients were discharged within one year of admission. Seven (17 per cent) had been readmitted by one year later. The average duration of stay was three months. We found no significant difference between men and women in this respect, and none between those who went home or into digs, hostels, and so on.

Thirty-three patients were discharged home, and the others went to live in digs, hostels, or elsewhere. Of the 7 patients readmitted, 4 were living at home and 3 were away from home. Again, we found no difference between the sexes in this respect.

Thirty-two patients were discharged to jobs. Twenty-six

[1] 24 per cent of all patients admitted to one of the hospitals during the period of the research were diagnosed as suffering from schizophrenia, paranoia, or paranoid states. This compares with the figures (also 24 per cent) available from the General Registrar Office for admissions in these three categories to hospitals in the North West Metropolitan Regional Area in 1958. Figures for later years are not yet published. Failure to state the criteria, clinical or social, on which diagnosis is based, and failure to give the percentage of admissions diagnosed as schizophrenic, render it impossible in many cases to evaluate reports on this subject.

worked for the whole year after discharge; two worked for less than a year but for more than six months. Once again, there was no significant difference between the sexes.

Twenty of the patients studied were first admissions, 13 men and 7 women. Of the 22 previous admissions, 7 were men and 15 women. Three of the 7 readmitted were first admissions, all women.

Patients readmitted* within a year of discharge

	No. discharged	No. readmitted	% readmitted
Men	20	2	10
Women	22	5	23
All Patients	42	7	17

* Readmitted means readmitted to any hospital or psychiatric unit. In fact none was readmitted elsewhere during the period in question.

Assessment

In general, the assessment of the results of psychiatric treatment presents great theoretical and methodological problems. This is particularly so with schizophrenia. No generally agreed method of assessing the results of treatment in schizophrenia exists, nor are there generally agreed indices of morbidity or criteria of cure.

The readmission rate is possibly the most widely used criterion of the continuing effectiveness of treatment, and a number of papers have been published in the U.S.A. using this criterion. They report widely varying readmission rates. A study on the use of chlorpromazine carried out by Tuteur (1959) showed that 20·4 per cent of patients discharged were back in hospital within three years, while Pollack (1958) in another study on chlorpromazine reported that, of 716 patients discharged, 19 per cent were readmitted. In a group treated with tranquillizers and monthly psychotherapeutic interviews, Mendel and Rapport (1963) found that 21·6 per cent were readmitted within one year. Free and Dodd (1961), in their study of 596 patients divided into a control and an after-care group, found that 3·51 per cent of the former and 14·6 per cent of the latter were back within a year of discharge. Recently Orlinski and D'Elia (1964) reported on 13,036 discharged schizophrenics and found that 45·5 per cent of those who received no after-care and 25·7 per cent of those who did were readmitted within a year.

Unfortunately, few comparable studies have been published in this country and there is no breakdown of relevant figures from the General Register Office.

A report by Renton *et al.* (1963) who followed up 132 men and women schizophrenics showed that 18 per cent were readmitted or had committed suicide within one year. While recently, Kelly and Sargant (1965) reporting on forty-eight schizophrenics of both sexes treated by various combinations of ECT, deep and modified insulin, and phenothiazines, show that, during a two-year follow-up, 42 per cent were readmitted at least once, and 6 per cent leucotomized. However, these two groups may not be comparable with ours. Apart from the fact that, for example, the group studied by Renton and her colleagues contains patients over sixty-five, sampling problems tend to make comparison difficult. In the case of the study by Kelly and Sargant, there is for instance, no account of the criteria for selection, and it does not appear that the diagnosis was checked by another psychiatrist independently or by consensus. In the report by Renton and her colleagues, the group studied was selected from among hospitalized patients whose recorded diagnosis came under Schizophrenic Disorders, number 300, ·0 to ·7 or Paranoia and Paranoid States, number 303 in the International Classification of Diseases. Those who met the researchers' diagnostic criteria were chosen on the basis of an examination of the case records. A number unspecified, all originally diagnosed on the basis of a clinical examination, were thus excluded. In addition it is not clear whether the decisions to exclude were checked by consensus or otherwise. Thus the group may not be representative of the patients normally diagnosed as schizophrenic in the hospital. This may have some bearing on the fact that the group included two suicides.

However, the Medical Research Council team at the Maudsley have published four papers which offer us certain points of comparison. Wing *et al.* (1959), in a report on a group of 158 schizophrenics admitted to a London hospital in 1955–6 and discharged within two years, showed that 19·4 per cent of the men and 30·9 per cent of the women were readmitted within two years of discharge. However, these figures applied only to readmissions to the same hospital. Another MRC report by Brown *et al.* (1961) showed among other things that, of 625 schizophrenic men and women admitted to three London mental hospitals in 1956 and discharged within two years, 64 per cent were readmitted in the three years following their key admissions.

More recently the same team (Brown *et al.*, 1962, Wing *et al.*, 1964) have reported on a group of male schizophrenics from eight London mental hospitals who were followed up for a year after discharge. Of 128 patients, 41 per cent (1962 study) were readmitted within the year. When the group was reduced (to 113) by excluding those about whose diagnosis the researchers had some doubt, the readmission rate remained substantially the same, 43 per cent (1964 study). However, these four studies, too, may not be strictly comparable with ours. For one reason, the MRC samples included people over the age of thirty-five, whereas ours did not.

The 1964 MRC study is in certain respects most suitable for the purposes of comparison, but again sampling problems make this difficult. For instance it is possible that their patients do not represent the persons diagnosed as schizophrenic by the hospital. Whereas the diagnosis of schizophrenia is established in our study by at least two psychiatrists independently within a short time of admission, in the MRC study (1964) the hospital diagnosis made at the time of admission when symptoms were presumably most marked was altered in 15 out of the 128 cases by one of the team who saw the patient for the first time just before discharge. This changed diagnosis was not checked by another psychiatrist and these fifteen patients were excluded from the final data.

We have discussed these difficulties with the MRC team, and

they have made a further analysis of their data, to provide a group as comparable as possible to ours as a discharge group. These figures have not yet been published, but the MRC team have kindly given us permission to reproduce them in this report. Taking the 1956 cohort (1961 report), they excluded those over thirty-five, and those who had stayed for more than one year in hospital, leaving 374 men and women, of whom 193 or 52 per cent were readmitted within the year. If this readmission group is sub-divided into men and women, and first and previous admissions, we find the following results.

Readmissions within one year, by first and previous admissions

	First admissions	% first admissions readmitted	Previous admissions	% previous admissions readmitted
Men	26	44	68	59
Women	30	42	69	56
All Patients	56	43	137	56

If we compare our results, as far as this is possible, with those quoted in the MRC studies, we find certain points of interest, although naturally we must be cautious about drawing final conclusions.

We cannot compare the readmission of men since the numbers of men readmitted in our sample is too low. However, comparing the total of men and women readmitted in our sample with the number of men reported readmitted in the MRC 1964 study, we find that 17 per cent of our patients were readmitted compared with 43 per cent of patients in the MRC study, and that this difference is statistically significant ($\chi^2 = 8 \cdot 34 \, p. < \cdot 005$).[1] Since the percentage of female readmissions in our study is more than twice that of males, this figure may well be weighted against us.

12 per cent of all patients in our group who were living at

[1] Yates correction used here.

		MRC STUDIES								OUR STUDY		
		1959 report (1955 cohort[1])		1961 report (1956 cohort)	1956 cohort personal communication			1962 report	1964 report	1964 report		
		men	women	all patients	men	women	all patients	men	men	men	women	all patients
1	size of cohort	123	75	715	—	—	—	not given	not given	20	22	42
2	No. of patients in discharge sample	103	55	625	176	198	374	128	113	20	22	42
3	% readmitted within one year	not given	not given	not given	53%	50%	52%	41%	43%	10%	23%	17%
4	% readmitted of those living at home	not given	not given	not given	—	—	—	45.7%	44.4%	6%	19%	12%
5	% readmitted of those living in digs, hostels, or with sibs	not given	not given	not given	—	—	—	29.4%	39.1%	33%	33%	33%
6	% working for more than half the time during the year after discharge	not given	not given	not given	—	—	—	not given	61.9%	80%	55%	67%
7	% working for whole of year after discharge	not given	not given	not given	—	—	—	not given	not given	70%	55%	62%
8	% first admissions in cohort discharged within 2 years of admission	93.5%	73.7%	91%	—	—	—	not given	not given	100%	100%	100%
9	% of previous admissions discharged within 2 years of key admission	77.9%	73.2%	86%	—	—	—	not given	not given	100%	100%	100%
10	% of cohort which are first admissions	37.4%	25.3%	33%	—	—	—	not given	not given	65%	32%	48%
11	% of discharge sample which are first admissions	not given	not given	not given	34%	36%	35%	not given	25.7%	65%	32%	48%
12	% of cohort under 35 years of age	52%	42.7%	not given	—	—	—	not given	not given	100%	100%	100%
13	Average age in years of cohort	not given	not given	not given	—	—	—	not given	not given	22.6	25.4	24.1
14	Average age in years of discharge sample	not given	not given	not given	—	—	—	not given	33.2	22.6	25.4	24.1

[1] Cohort means cohort in key admission

home were readmitted, compared with 44·4 per cent (men only) readmitted of those living at home in the group reported in the MRC 1964 study. However, the total number of our patients readmitted is less than five and so our figure cannot be regarded as statistically significant although a trend emerges ($x^2 = 8·99$ $p. < 005$).[1]

Discussion

In this report we do not claim that our approach to the problem of schizophrenia is the only one possible, or even the best. We are primarily concerned to show that this form of family-orientated social therapy which has been relatively neglected in this country is at least effective. We are thus less interested in paring down percentage figures than in showing that our results compare favourably with those reported for other methods.

In respect of readmission rate, our figures appear to be statistically considerably less than the national trend in so far as that trend can be assessed. It might be suggested that the reason why so few of our patients returned to hospital was because of improved community care services (after-care hostels, etc.). In fact only two of our patients were discharged to hostels. All the others returned home or went into lodgings. In all cases we provided the after-care which was an extension of family therapy and consisted essentially in our being available for consultation whenever the family, the patient, or the general practitioners felt the need. The average number of consultations per family in the year after discharge was three. These ranged from telephone conversations to full family discussion. Brown *et al.* report (1962) a significant tendency for patients who return to homes where there is high emotional involvement with a key relative to be readmitted more frequently. Of the five women readmitted, two were not living with their families, and of the two men readmitted, one was living away from his family.

As for the condition of the patients who were not readmitted, 72 per cent of the men and 70 per cent of the women were

---

[1] Yates correction used here.

capable of a sufficient social adjustment to be able to earn their living for the whole of the year after discharge.

The trends are clear. Schizophrenics now 'remit' quite quickly in hospital. Most of them, however, have to return to the social context in which they broke down in the first place. In most cases this social context is the family of origin. At least 50 per cent of first-admission schizophrenics who return to their family of origin are back in hospital within one year (as far as the national trend can be assessed). The figure rises as emotional involvement with any key member of the family becomes more intense.

For socio-economic reasons, for a long time to come patients will have to go back to their families and they will have to put up with one another. We try to help the patient and his family to be less disturbing to each other by intensive work with the whole family including the patient during his stay in hospital. By the time the patient is discharged they have perhaps learned to understand one another a little better and come to feel there is someone else who understands them. They are encouraged to feel that in any crisis they can refer back to us for an emergency family consultation either at hospital or, where hospital arrangements have allowed, *in their own home*. In the last five years these forty-two families have called us out seven times in all. We arranged readmission on two occasions. The patient would probably have been rehospitalized on three of the other five occasions under usual circumstances. Of the remaining five cases readmitted, one was a woman who needed hostel accommodation but was readmitted because none was immediately available, and four were hospitalized without our knowledge. This was because we had to work within a hospital O.P. and domiciliary service in which (i) a psychiatrist unknown to the patient may see him on a routine visit to the O.P. department, (ii) the family is usually never seen at all, and (iii) the psychiatrist, if called on a domiciliary visit, has no knowledge of the family and has no time to acquire any.

Summary

Twenty male and twenty-two female schizophrenics were treated by conjoint family and milieu therapy in two mental hospitals, with reduced use of tranquillizers. No individual psychotherapy was given. None of the so-called shock treatments was given, nor was leucotomy. All patients were discharged within one year of admission. The average length of stay was three months. Seventeen per cent were readmitted within one year of discharge. Seventy per cent of those not readmitted were able to earn their livings for the whole of the year after discharge. Our results are discussed. They appear to us to establish at least a prima facie case for radical revision of the therapeutic strategy employed in most psychiatric units in relation to the schizophrenic and his family. This revision is in line with current developments in social psychiatry in the United Kingdom.

Acknowledgements

We are grateful to the consultant psychiatrists at the hospitals concerned for their co-operation in enabling this work to be carried out, and to the clinical and nursing staffs of both hospitals, whose help was, of course, invaluable.

We would also like to thank the following for their helpful criticism and advice on the preparation of this paper: Dr E. J. M. Bowlby, Dr G. W. Brown, Professor G. M. Carstairs, Dr C. M. Parkes, Dr J. H. Patterson, and Professor T. Ferguson Rodger.

References to Appendix

BATESON, G., JACKSON, D. D., HALEY, J. & WEAKLAND, J. (1956). Toward a theory of schizophrenia. *Behav. Sci.* **1**, 251.

BROWN, G. W., PARKES, C. M. & WING, J. K. (1961). Admissions and readmissions to three mental hospitals. *J. Ment. Sci.* **107**, 1070–7.

BROWN, G. W., MONCK, E. M., CARSTAIRS, G. M. & WING, J. K. (1962). Influence of family life on the course of schizophrenic illness. *Brit. J. prev. soc. Med.* **16**, 55.

FREE, S. & DODD, D. (1961). Aftercare for discharged mental

patients: conference on a five-state study of mental health in Virginia. 11, 28.

KELLY, D. H. W. & SARGANT, W. (1965). Present treatment of schizophrenia – a controlled follow-up study. *Brit. med. J.* (1), 147–50.

KREITMAN, N. (1961). The reliability of psychiatric diagnosis. *J. Ment. Sci.* **107**, 876–86.

LAING, R. D. & ESTERSON, A. (1964). *Sanity, madness, and the family.* Volume I, *Families of schizophrenics.* London: Tavistock Publications; New York: Basic Books.

LIDZ, T., CORNELISON, A., TERRY, D. & FLECK, S. (1958). Intrafamilial environment of the schizophrenic patient. VI The transmission of irrationality. *AMA Archives of Neurology and Psychiatry* **79**, 305–16.

MENDEL, W. M., & RAPPORT, S. (1963). Outpatient treatment for chronic schizophrenic patients. *Arch. Gen. Psychiat.* **8**, 190.

ORLINEKI, N. & D'ELIA, E. (1964). Rehospitalisation of the schizophrenic patient. *Arch. Gen. Psychiat.* **10**, 47–54.

POLLACK, B. (1958). The effect of chlorpromazine in reducing the relapse rate in 716 released patients. *Amer. J. Psychiat.* **114**, 749.

RENTON, C. A., AFFLECK, J. W., CARSTAIRS, G. M. & FORREST, A. D. (1963). A follow-up of schizophrenic patients in Edinburgh. *Acta psychiat. scand.* **39**, 548–81.

TUTEUR, W., STILLER, R. & GLOTZER, J. (1959). Discharged mental hospital chlorpromazine patients. *Diseases of the Nervous System* **20**, 512.

WING, J. K., DENHAM, J. & MONRO, A. B. (1959). Duration of stay in hospital of patients suffering from schizophrenia. *Brit. J. prev. soc. Med.* **13**, 145–8.

WING, J. K., MONCK, E. BROWN, G. W. & CARSTAIRS, G. M. (1964). Morbidity in the community of schizophrenic patients discharged from London mental hospital in 1959. *Brit. J. Psychiat.* **110**, 10–21.

WYNNE, L. C., RYCKOFF, I. M., DAY, J. & HIRSCH, S. (1958). Pseudomutuality in the family relations of schizophrenics. *Psychiatry* **21**, 205.

References

ARIES, P. (1960). *L'Enfant et la vie familiale sous l'Ancien Régime.* Paris: Plon.

ARTISS, KENNETH L. (1962). *Milieu therapy in schizophrenia.* New York: Grune & Stratton.

BATESON, G., JACKSON, D. D., HALEY, J. & WEAKLAND, J. (1956). Toward a theory of schizophrenia. *Behav. Sci.* I, 251.

BETTELHEIM, B. (1961). *The informed heart.* London: Thames & Hudson.

BOWEN, M. (1959). Family relationships. In Alfred Auerback (ed.), *Schizophrenia: an integrated approach.* New York: Ronald Press.

GIBRAN, K. (1926). *The prophet.* London: Heinemann.

GOLDSTEIN, K. (1951). *Die Aufbau des Organismus.* The Hague: M. Nijhoff, 1934.

IONESCO, E. (1950). *The bald prima donna.* London: Calder, 1958.

JONES, MAXWELL (1952). *Social psychiatry.* London: Tavistock Publications. Under the title *The therapeutic community*, New York: Basic Books, 1954.

LAING, R. D. (1960). *The divided self.* London: Tavistock Publications (also Harmondsworth: Penguin Books, 1965).

— (1961). *The self and others.* London: Tavistock Publications.

LAING, R. D. & COOPER, D. G. (1964). *Reason and violence.* London: Tavistock Publications; New York: Humanities Press.

LAING, R. D. & ESTERSON, A. (1964). *Sanity, madness, and the family.* Volume I, *Families of schizophrenics.* London: Tavistock Publications; New York: Basic Books.

LÉVI-STRAUSS, C. (1953). Social structure. In A. L. Kroeber (ed.), *Anthropology today.* Chicago: University of Chicago Press.

— (1955). *Tristes Tropiques.* Paris: Plon.

ROSENFELD, H. (1955). Psycho-analysis of the super-ego conflict in an acute schizophrenic patient. In M. Klein, P. Heimann, and R. Money-Kyrle (eds.), *New directions in psycho-analysis*. London: Tavistock Publications; New York: Basic Books.

RUSSELL, B. (1913). *Principia mathematica*.

SARTRE, J.-P. (1943). *L'Être et le néant*. Paris. (English translation by H. E. Barnes, *Being and nothingness*. London: Methuen, 1957).

SARTRE, J.-P. (1952). *Saint Genet. Comédien et martyr*. Paris: Gallimard.

SARTRE, J.-P. (1957). *Being and nothingness*. Translated by H. E. Barnes. London: Methuen.

SARTRE, J.-P. (1960). *Critique de la raison dialectique*. Paris: Gallimard.

SZASZ, T. S. (1962). *The myth of mental illness*. London: Secker and Warburg.

WEAKLAND, J. H. (1960). The 'double-bind' hypothesis of schizophrenia and three-party interaction. In D. D. Jackson (ed.), *The etiology of schizophrenia*. New York: Basic Books.

WILMER, HARRY A. (1958). *Social psychiatry in action*. Springfield, Ill.: C. C. Thomas.

WYNNE, L. C., RYCKOFF, I. M., DAY, J. & HIRSCH, S. (1958). Pseudomutuality in the family relations of schizophrenics. *Psychiatry* **21**, 205.